I've Never Been an Old Man

What it's Like if You Plan to Age

Don Larsen

Foreword by
Dr. Grace Devnich

ACTIVE BOOKS

I've Never Been an Old Man
Don Larsen

Copyright © 2004 by Active Books. All rights reserved. No part of this book may be reproduced in any form, or by any means, except for the inclusion of brief quotations for review purposes, without prior written permission of the author.

First printing April 2004

Library of Congress Control Number: 2003114749

ISBN 0-9746675-4-4

Printed in U.S.A. by Mennonite Press, Inc., Newton, KS 67114

Foreword

Don shows with humor how to conquer the stress of care giving with humor and the assistance of three female felines. The book is upbeat in spite of a bumpy road for he and Jacquie, his wife. While the bits of wit and love between the chuckholes in the road of life have helped the couple, the reader can also benefit from his story.

*Dr. Grace Devnich**

---

*Dr. Devnich is an inspiration to those fortunate to know her. At ninety-one she published a biography about her mother-in-law coming from Russia as a single lady to homestead in South Dakota. Now at ninety-six, she is writing of her father who started formal education at eighteen and earned a medical degree at thirty. This spring she attended a medical conference in Southern California and enrolled in several classes.

Dedicated to Jacqueline J. Hawbecker,
the girl I courted

The woman who became my wife

The lady I call
"My JJL"

Special Thanks

I wish to thank a number of people making the last two years less of a problem than they could have been. Thanks to Penny, our insurance agent, for providing guidance to financially cope with our trials. Lori, we thank you for helping locate the Chateau, which serves Jacquie so well. Doctor Banda, you deserve many thanks for guiding us healthwise for many years. Not only are you our doctor, you are our friend. Sue and Maribec, you have made the Chateau a real home for Jacquie. Not only does our HMO, Kaiser Permanente, deserve credit for top service but their hospital in Walnut Creek is an example of an institution dedicated to service to clients in an award winning manner. I also appreciate the night clerks at Safeway and the Realtors at marketing meetings who greet me with concern about my wife who they do not know but out of interest in both of us. Many who had been sole caretakers warned me to be careful of stress due to their personal experiences. I am impressed by the demonstration of the humanism of the human race.

Beth Brewster, Arlene Folkers, Ruth Gasten, Barbara Gilson, Margaret Lucke, Marilou Mazetti, Nancy O'Connell, Ann Peters, and Penny Warren your assistance with words made this retelling possible.

Thanks
Don

Table of Contents

Part One...Before it Happened

Chapter 1 A Frightening Awakening / I'm Making Luck* 7

Chapter 2 Adoption-Adaptation, Who Adopted and
Adopted to Whom?/Four Feet and Whiskers 17

Chapter 3 Another HMO Adventure / JJL is MIA at the HMO 29

Chapter 4 Our October of Life Sub-plots / My Three Falls,
But I'm Not Out 37

Chapter 5 Fiasco at the Doctor's Office / Where did
the 12 IVs go? 45

Chapter 6 My Second Sweetheart / Programmed by the Cats . 57

Chapter 7 Senior Sitting, Napping and Illness / I Can't
Nap with Three Females 65

Chapter 8 A Poor Start Indeed! / Things Change, I love it! 73

Chapter 9 Rather Than Talk, They Wrote Me /
It's Your Turn the Letter Said 85

Chapter 10 Life Returns Today / I Have
Communication Glitches 93

Chapter 11 I lost my Right Ear last Night / Hospital Hi-jinks .. 99

Chapter 12 A Lull Between ER Visits / I am my Own Assessor . 109

Chapter 13 What About Other Cancers / Karen, Our Dynamo . 115

* Sub-titles.

Chapter 14 Relax While You Can, Don / How Do you Plan
for What's Ahead? 121

Chapter 15 "911 and 911 Again" / Togetherness on 580 and 680   125

Chapter 16 She Listens With her Mouth / I Just Miss
the ER Room 131

Chapter 17 Valves, Dizziness and Drizzles / Why Should
I Live so Long? 135

Chapter 18 My October Sky Rockets / Wet Noise 143

Chapter 19 Am I Going Down for the Count? / Aging can
Mean Mature Confusion 147

Chapter 20 Blue Moon Halloween / The Quiet Before it
Comes Apart 155

Chapter 21 Sitting? No! Sitting With a Reason /
Am I Changing? 163

Chapter 22 She Does it Again but Head First This Time! /
"Oh No, Jacquie!" 167

Chapter 23 Never go Barefoot in Second Childhood /
The Stage is Being Set Again 173

Chapter 24 Good Morning, or is it? / Some Mornings
can be Hectic 179

Chapter 25 An Old Nemesis, 911, Again / An HMO Christmas   185

Part Two...Now We Part

Chapter 26 We Must Leave Each Other / Today's the Day! 197

Chapter 27 End of a Part of My Life / JJL and I Start Over 209

Chapter 28 Together, We Live Alone! / By Darn,
Let's Make it Work! 215

Part Three...Now We Know

Chapter 29 Now We Know / Four Months Later 227

Chapter 30 The Weekend Date / She is Home Again 235

Chapter 31 Can We Celebrate This One? / Fifty-five or Bust ... 241

Chapter 32 I Talk Back to the Judge / Cat Husbandry
            With No Degree 249

Chapter 33 Fainting and Slipping in the Shower /
            I Can't Call 911 257

Chapter 34 The Day of the Female / A Miniature Prim Lady ... 265

Chapter 35 Thoughts and Re-Thoughts / I Get Away With It .. 269

Chapter 36 After Hours Peep Shows / Early Morning Beauties . 275

Chapter 37 Oh No, Not Again! / Will We Learn to
            Avoid Calling 911? 281

Preface

The authors of mysteries, romances and most adventure stories have at least one destination or goal they work toward as they progress through their work: the mystery is solved, the courtship leads to marriage or the mountain is reached. The destination at the end of a journey is quite important. However, not all journeys in life end like this. The purpose of a Sunday afternoon ride may be simply to enjoy the journey.

I am enjoying cruising through the last trimester of my life. I definitely am in my October with November on the next calendar page. I strongly disagree with the concept that one should put aside the active for the inactive life upon retirement. I write to emphasize that point. Get in; buckle your seat belt as I enjoy some of my golden years, our cats, health misfortunes and anything else crossing the highway of my life.

I just heard the traffic forecast and its not good. There's a road closure, several 911 calls, with firepersons and medics just several miles ahead.

Full speed ahead!

A counselor for the New York Fire Department states all individuals have one or more Ground Zero experiences: a child killed, a divorce, losing a home or the passing of parents. Our Ground Zero is just down the road a bit and will last for the rest or our journey.

Part One
Before It Happened

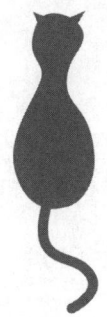

Author's Statement

When you're over the hill, life can be different. The scenery may change, as does the road map. There may be new bumps in the road and road names may no longer sound familiar. Everyone's freeway leads towards the township called Aging. People my age usually had a grandparent no longer able to live alone living with their children, our parents. We children learned about aging daily. Rosie the Riveter laid down her rivet gun after the second world not to care for parents but to work downtown. Her children, the Baby Boomers, had little chance to observe their grandparents aging as they were in rest homes.

Jacquie and I were enjoying the Highway of Life until we finished out fifty-fourth anniversary brunch. At that moment we met a detour and our lives changed forever. After Jacquie's many trips to the emergency room, the hospital and my ambulance trips, it was decided on Christmas Day in a hospital room that Jacquie should live in a rest home. We were fortunate to find a good home. Doctors and neighbors tell us we are now doing better and look healthier.

This story cannot be classified as a romance. It is a love story or better said, a story with a lot of emotion. Care giving is a gift of love. This sharing is not limited to us as a couple. The members of my harem, Latte, Mocha and Java, three female cats, receive and return a lot of feeling. Their purring, rubbing against legs or licking a wrist helps lower my stress level.

Besides the coffee cats there are two other important characters in this eighteen-month tale. One was also born on my day of birth. I call this inner voice, Self. We do a lot of conversing and arguing that no one else hears. Sergeant Sue, Jacquie's caretaker, has become a close friend.

I am an optimist with a goodly amount of humor. While we have problems, Self and I manage to perceive little things that are positive and often humorous. Being ill is not funny but some humor can be found in most situations.

"How old is old?" Self, my inner companion and antagonist since birth, asks from behind my ear. By his tone and the way he asks his question, I know he is going to taunt me for awhile so I need to be careful with any answers.

"When talking about aging you deal in years with wine, guarantees and car models but with people it's different. It's a relative thing. Some women think they're old at thirty and stop quoting their age. Many employees think they're old when close to retirement. Age depends on many factors, especially the attitude of the person. One of the most active minds I know belongs to a ninety six-year old lady doctor, Dr. Grace D. She lives alone, drives and uses a computer to write books. She has just published one about her mother-in-law coming from southern Russia to homestead land in frontier North Dakota. She's now writing a history of her parents. She left class early Tuesday to go to Southern California to a medical conference where she's signed up for classes.

When I was a kid we knew anyone sixty was a very old person. Now that I'm past that age marker, I think it is interesting to talk about what life is about beyond the sixties. Now I'm almost through the seventies so current happenings are my topic. Is life different in the seventies?"

"Where I sit up here on your shoulder, it appears that there is life for some of you old timers Don, although I see many that are not as fortunate."

'Thanks, smart alec.' I believe I make most of my luck and that also goes for the life I'm able to live. I think that's the reason wineries work in aging cellars to make grape juice into vintage wines. I'm hoping to have a few vintage experiences yet. I need to keep things going strong to be able to be a supportive spouse to my unfortunate wife. If I don't, I'll sour like bad wine."

"I didn't think I can win any argument with you, Don, as you don't always pay attention to your conscience. But thanks for listening."

"Thanks for your candor. Your questions caused me to think of several things I want to address in the chapters ahead."

"Any you can share with this old buddy?"

"One hint, the number of years is not as important as the quality of the life one has lived."

"I get it. Your Jacquie is living more days but the quality of her days are not as good as they were or could be."

"Exactly."

"Your family appreciates you for trying to put more quality into her days even though she's at a rest home. Your son, Larry complimented you for that on Father's Day. Remember? I appreciate being your sidekick! Now Don, retell the story of your last two years."

Chapter 1

A Frightening Awakening
I'm Making Luck

I awaken with my nightly emergency. I jump out of bed as quickly as I can move at my age, replacing the covers to keep our bed warm. Then I do a quick shuffle to the master bathroom. I don't need a light. We built the house decades ago and I know the way. I've been to the bathroom many times.

Several years ago, I reached that select age when senior men awaken in the middle of the night. Avoiding drinking liquids after dinner has not solved my problem completely, as an emergency call can still come sometime between 2:45 and 6:15. The bathroom clock is proclaiming 3:58 in large red digital numerals, readable without my glasses. These clocks are a necessity if geriatric folks want to check the time in the middle of the night.

Seeing the clock as I start for the little room reminds me of a morning several weeks ago – another time when I had to get up in the night. I had to arise at five to take our daughter to the hospital for cancer tests. The night before, my wife, Jacquie, or JJL as I call her, asked, "Are you going to set the alarm?"

"No, I'll drink a glass of water at bedtime, and use my internal alarm," I replied. I had a big glass of water, and Karen and I made the appointment with time to spare.

At my age, having to get up in the night does not bother me. In fact, I am quite glad to be around to experience septuagenarian problems. If you're laid out in your sixties, you'll never know what you could have enjoyed later. It's better to become a septuagenarian than the alternative, not becoming one! As a child six decades ago, I knew that anyone in his or her sixties was a very old person indeed. We kids considered such people to be relics beyond their time. Exceeding my childhood expectations by at least a decade is very satisfying. I'm now shooting to exceed my earlier goals by two decades or more. "Life has been good to me," I tell Self, that inner part of me hidden from everyone else.

"You're right," Self replies on a channel that only I can receive.

I like it when Self agrees with me. I'm not sleepy and continue, "Not only that, I'm still in good health and very active. Hallelujah!" Seniors, even people in general, don't "hallelujah" enough between aches and other problems. We need to look for plusses to celebrate, even little plusses or gains. It's good therapy for the soul and quite inexpensive, I tell myself as I pet Mocha, my cat, who's arisen from her bed to join me in the bathroom. She supervises my activities and hopes to gain some petting. She teases me by rubbing her soft coat against my bare leg and I succumb to her wishes. Hallelujah for an early morning friend!

The real worry as I crawl back into my still warm bed is, "Can I get back to sleep?" I manage to return to sleep only about one time out of four, which is a poor batting average. I have an active brain. It becomes refreshed hours before my body and it enjoys getting the day started early with lots of random thoughts and planning.

This habit of mental activity probably developed due to the boredom I endured while riding a mule-drawn row-crop cultivator as a boy in the Midwest. Farm boys were expected to carry their weight early in life, and cultivating corn was one way a young child could help out. It was a lonely job. The rows of corn were a quarter or a half-mile long, which meant the round trip to the far side of the field and back was a half-mile or a mile. The mule time for the trip on a hot June day was considerable, leaving a lot of time for this dusty boy to daydream or wonder. The cultivator seat was slung low between the tall wheels so the operator's feet could guide the shovels toward or away from the young corn plants. With the corn shoulder high on each side, and only the rumps of the mules close ahead and towering above me, the scenery was minimal at best. There was little other sensual input, no interesting sounds, only the smell of the freshly turned soil and the temperature of the air as it turned from chilly at dawn, to a warm midday, to downright hot in the afternoon. These sensual inputs lost their impact after several miles of slow riding. It was on these days that Self and I became quite well acquainted and developed the easy habit of sharing thoughts.

While my mind daydreamed, this tow-headed boy did develop a skill or two. I learned to estimate distance and its relationship to time: "I'm halfway back, and it should take another fifteen minutes. Then I'll get the water jug from under the thorny hedge trees surrounding the field and have a drink." Thinking of the cool water in the glass gallon jug wrapped in a wet gunnysack seemed to make the distance and the time go even slower and my thirst increase. It was a dirty place down there between the wheels and near the shovels stirring up dust. There was seldom any breeze to blow the dust away or cool me. Certainly the mules weren't going fast enough to create a breeze. Their tails switching the giant horseflies did little to stir the air, either. A horsefly drilling for blood would excite a horse but the mules just switched their tails faster.

Crawling back into bed after my bathroom respite this morning, I vow to keep from thinking about anything that would cause me to stay awake. "I will pull a shade down in front of my mind so everything will go blank. I should be asleep in five minutes," I tell Self.

"Want'a bet?" Self teases.

The shade doesn't work, so I concentrate on counting to myself: "One thousand one, one thousand two, one thousand three." When I get to, "one thousand twenty-nine," I realize my carefully conceived numerical battle campaign has been defeated. The scheming portion of my mind has outflanked the go-to-sleep portion and won the war.

"Shall I go for a walk before leaving at seven for the Realtors' meeting in Walnut Creek or shall I go to the computer for some word processing?" I ask myself.

"You don't have enough January dawn before your seven o'clock departure to go for a long walk." Self has done the arithmetic. I get up, shave, dress for the day, and go to the microwave to heat instant coffee.

My plan is greatly modified by the senior Siamese cat, Latte. She is endowed with managerial and administrative attributes, and being female, she commandeers priority one. She hops from her sleeping position on JJL's thighs, and follows me to the kitchen. I spot her as I reach for my cup. She sits in a conspicuous spot and looks into my eyes. Though she is silent, her eyes state, "I'm ready for breakfast. Get with it, master!"

Fifteen minutes later, with headlights on, my little GMC and I skirt downtown Livermore and head west, away from the developing sunrise of the new day. I soon find myself the last in a long line of cars with red taillights. "Why do I sit in a half-mile backup waiting to get onto the 580 freeway where commute traffic is all but stopped?" I ask Self.

"It's the same every morning," Self reminds me. "You've driven this for years. You shouldn't be surprised."

After several miles of slow driving I pass the golf course and traffic speeds up. Highway 680 going north will be faster but also crowded. I can go the twenty-five miles in forty-five minutes. And I do this for what? To chat with Realtors as I hand them the word-search puzzles I create in the hope they will remember to use our family's house-inspection business when their clients buy a house. "Is it worth all the trouble and stress?" I often ask our son Jon. "The puzzles don't get inspection orders." Jon replies, "They insure the inspection firm's name is remembered, at least until the puzzle has been finished later in the day. Even the people who don't take a puzzle remember us."

Stationing myself inside the entrance to their meeting, I greet the first arrival, "Good morning. You're looking healthy and wearing a pretty smile this morning."

She smiles. "I am well. What's the puzzle about this week, Don?" She remembers my name and I am pleased. My marketing is working. She'll also remember our company's name.

"Obituaries."

"Are you kidding?"

"Nope. I included the words New Year's resolutions, Christmas cards, 49er Super Bowl chances, post-Christmas sales and 33-cent postage stamps. These things all died on or before New Year's Day, hence the title Obituaries."

"OK. I always make a copy of your puzzles to send to my granddaughter. You have software that helps you make the puzzles, don't you?"

"Yes."

The next person is a man unknown to me. When offered a puzzle he replies, "I'm not smart enough for that stuff."

"Instead of smarts, these word-search puzzles rely upon perception," I counter. "We develop this skill in the fellows we trained as inspectors. We had to teach them to perceive what others saw but did not perceive. That describes our inspection business." As an artist, I've learned a lot about the importance of perception. I notice the grass varies from a yellow-green nearby to a blue-green in the distance. The sky at the horizon is a different blue than the blue overhead.

I hand this Realtor a business card instead of a puzzle.

"Well, thanks. Now I better get my coffee and a doughnut," he states as he moves toward the serving table.

Forty minutes after I arrive, the meeting is starting. I have handed out thirty or forty puzzles at this, the first of three meetings I will attend this week. I will have a new puzzle for the meetings next week. After the flag salute I slip out of the room by the back door to retrieve my truck. It is parked near the parking lot entrance where it is the first logo the Realtors see as they arrive. Buckling my seatbelt, and sipping the coffee I didn't have time to drink while talking with the Realtors, I guide my little white chariot onto the route home. My wandering mind begins one of the many journeys it will traverse today.

"Poor old Clarence," I say to Self, thinking back to the last person I gave a puzzle to. This little man has a bad curvature of the spine.

Self observes, "He is becoming more stooped as he ages, yet he is quite alert. I like him. I'll bet he's seventy-eight or eighty if he's a day, but his countenance says sixty or thereabouts."

Clarence arrived late today, so bypassed the puzzle for a change as he headed for the coffee bar. He gave me a broad smile and a nod of his balding head, as he does to everyone. I'm not sure if he is active in the real estate market or just helps his daughter run the office. He was at a house, which our son Jon inspected last week. Whether Clarence uses a license any more or just helps her I don't know. Either way, it is important for him to keep busy to avoid a lot of the hazards and snares of aging.

My silent companion confirms my thoughts, "I believe an active mind and body retards the aging process."

"Use it or lose it," was the theme of Charles Osgood's little bit on the radio earlier in the week. He quoted research finding the game of Bingo to be useful in helping the mind retain its function and ability. I saw a pitch for an on-line university that said attitude and motivation are the keys to keeping the mind active and learning.

I wonder how many years I can maintain my pace, attending three marketing meetings in two counties every week and producing a monthly newsletter and distributing several thousand copies of it in a dozen towns. "I'm seventy-five, going for seventy-six and shooting for eighty," I vow.

"Seeing and talking to people is good preventive medicine for you," Self asserts as if he has a counseling degree. "Perhaps it's Common Sense 101."

"Good for Clarence too. Good for all of us," I say aloud. "Keeping active is not only good for the body; it is essential for the soul." I've tried to stay active mentally and physically. Maybe that's the reason people underestimate my age. I've got to get back to my watercolors and resume my artistic work. I want to go out of this life with a paintbrush in my hand. I want be a glorious splash of color in people's memories! I need to create some hallelujahs for others.

Self encourages me, "You can't be Grandma Moses, but you can be Grandpa Larsen."

"I believe computers, e-mail and chat rooms are positives for seniors if they will accept them," I tell Self. "The silicon miracles are a great way to keep the mind agile and alert when the body is beginning to lose its stamina. I'm lucky I can still write and distribute our newsletter. Marketing meetings give me a reason to arise and meet people in a meaningful manner. Most agents are younger than I am, and that's good company for me to keep. I have the respect of friends, something we all need, especially seniors."

Self agrees. "I'm worried that our country may have an epidemic of neglected elderly persons if we're not careful. Too often, meaningful associations with others are forgotten."

"A radio commentator addressed the issue last week," I remind him. He said that too many people disconnect with life when they retire." This is part of what ails my wife. She withdrew from life and became a recluse two decades ago. I was to learn in several weeks that JJL's serious problems would worsen and change our lives forever. The opportunity to make new friends often lessens as one moves from the freshman decade of senior citizenship, through its sophomore and junior stages, and beyond.

"Don," Self reminds me, "you've always said you believe you make most of your luck, both good and bad, and that the process must continue into the senior years."

"Yes, I can have a lot to do with my luck," I say.

I remember the little communities in the mid west where I grew up. Farmers would move to the villages when the time came to enjoy their retirement. But without the demands of a busy life, their minds or bodies suffered, and they died within a few years, leaving a community of farm widows. Housekeeping chores, church work and other hobbies gave the women a purpose, and they outlived husbands by a number of years. "Life must have a purpose," I conclude. "We must have, or develop, a purpose to enjoy our later lives."

Stopping at the last light before the freeway near nine A.M., I remember my plans for my senior years. I will retire from one activity to a less demanding one, but always one with something of a challenge. My watercolors can take me to my last day. I am slowing down; I do not go to as many meetings of the four art societies I support as I once did. I still judge four or five county fair art shows each summer without a hitch, but I enter fewer juried shows each year.

I recall a fellow school administrator's statement, "My Frank came home after his last day's work, hung up his hat and retired permanently to his chair. He hasn't moved to mow the lawn, help me around the house or take up a hobby." Life is much too short for that sort of retirement and that kind of inactivity isn't good for anyone. I'm keyed up on this concept. Retirement is a time to live, not rust and rot!

It is time to off-ramp the freeway and place newsletters in Realtor mailboxes in Danville. If I hurry I will get this done and still arrive at my junior-college writing class in time for a senior bathroom break. "Years ago," I confide to Self, "I got more than a hundred miles to a cup of coffee. Now it's only about fifty on the best of days. I wonder if my bladder is shrinking or just losing its elasticity. Now to save stops on long trips, instead of drinking coffee with caffeine to stay awake, I chew several strong mints."

My live-in philosopher reminds me, "A minute saved is a minute gained. Your senior minutes become more valuable each day."

I retort, "I intend for my minutes to have a purpose. If they have purpose there will be more of them; that's what I believe. As I told you earlier, I believe I make a lot of my luck. Purposeful minutes are my goal. Without purpose, minutes are not life."

Back onto the freeway, I listen to the traffic report. There is so much traffic in the San Francisco Bay area that most news stations post traffic reports every ten minutes. There are no problems where I'm going, but that is not true for everyone. There is a ladder in a lane on a nearby road. I hear of rolls of carpet, ladders, water heaters, and other strange obstacles on the highway quite often. I feel grateful for the cell phones many commuters carry. They are able to report road conditions to the radio stations so the rest of us can be warned.

My Tuesday morning writing class has too many of us for one session, but the college does not want to break the group into two. We read for five minutes, but Nancy, the instructor, is able to make only spelling or punctuation corrections on the copies we hand her. There is no chance for her to give more substantial feedback. However, the class is a great activity for us seniors. Some classmates are in their eighties, and several are in their tenth decade of life, the nineties. Many have college degrees and many do not. Most use computers and a few are of the yellow pad persuasion. One senior lady who started life in a non English-speaking family has just won another national writing prize. We each have our own purpose for writing, even if it's just to find enjoyment in the process. The class gives us motivation. Sharing is the frosting on the cake. Without the class the writing might be postponed.

On the way home I buy a hot dog without onions for JJL. I tell friends, "Jacquie has petitioned God to recall all members of the onion family, including garlic and chives; but God in Her wisdom apparently pigeonholed the request." I think the garlic and onion growers must pray to God to subsidize their bulbs, as I cannot find frozen food that doesn't contain them. To lose some weight, I will have cottage cheese and a head of Romaine lettuce for lunch.

Before stepping through the door between the garage and the kitchen, I know what I will find. My cat, Mocha, having heard the automatic garage door cranking open, will be sitting on a dining room chair near the door, waiting for some petting. Feeling her soft coat and hearing her purring probably does as much for me as the petting does for her. Hallelujah! Her fur feels like the refined silk of an oriental potentate. Next an arm will reach above JJL's recliner, which faces the other direction toward the TV. Two of Jacquie's fingers will be extended. She too has heard the door opener in spite the loudness of the TV. The high volume of the TV informs me she is not wearing her hearing aids. As per the finger request, (or is it an order?) I deliver two acetaminophen capsules and a glass of water. I know her headache is with her again today.

I also know what I'll see as I round the recliner with the medication. Latte, Jacquie's dark Siamese cat, is asleep, stretched between her mistress's knees. Not wanting to disturb this miniature family member, Jacquie continued suffering her headache until I arrived home. JJL has several routine medications that cause drowsiness. As a result, she can sleep several hours in the morning, afternoon, evening or all of the above. Latte, needs her species' eighteen hours of sleep. She keeps a close watch to see if her mistress is going to nap on the bed or in the recliner. If JJL iis not in either place the beautiful Siamese naps in a toweled basket or a cloth-hooded cat bed in the sun.

"Jacquie, why didn't you put Latte in my recliner and go for headache pills?"

"I don't want to disturb her sleep. Would you like to have your dreams disturbed?"

"Was she dreaming again?"

"Was she! An hour ago she suddenly jumped eighteen inches into the air and landed beside the recliner with eyes wide, hair erect on her back and a fluffy tail. I have a three-inch scratch on my right thigh and blood spots on my nightie and robe. It wasn't a dream: it was a nightmare."

"Whatever caused that nickel-sized wound she had on her hip when we adopted her must have been traumatic," I reply. "It remains in her subconscious memory. I can't solve her nightmare problems, but I can help you at headache time when she's on your lap."

"How? You're never around when I need you!"

I sense unhappiness. "Shift into careful gear," Self warns me.

I get a bottle of acetaminophen and place it on the end table by her recliner. "Here," I say. "You always seem to have iced tea here, and you can use it to take the pain killer." I sometimes believe I'm a second-class nurse. I know I am becoming a needed nurse more often.

"In spite of your doctor's best care, your wife's health is not better, and is starting to slip downward," Self whispers.

Jacquie says, "Don, you're always at the computer or in the bathroom working puzzles, rather than here beside me like a husband when I need you." I am right to be careful. Not feeling well, she likes to sit in her recliner. When awake, she watches TV. In the evenings, and if I'm not interested in her program I can sometimes get away with reading an English mystery. Is this retirement? For too many people a sedentary life is their idea of retirement. Life often deals a strange deck of cards. TV is not a priority on my list of important activities. I tune the TV set to a music channel, with no picture, as I write or do housework when JJL sleeps.

Reading my thoughts, Self concurs. "To each his own."

Before becoming ill, Jacquie enjoyed carding, dying, spinning and weaving wool into garments and art objects. She was not sedentary then. She was also challenged when running, via our fax machine, The Open Door, a gift store in Kansas. I have priorities other than tube-watching, but being wanted as an accomplice to TV-watching is not too bad. We all need to be needed. Sometimes, with my head turned toward the TV I script my plans for writing or painting. Then I might hear, "Are you asleep, Don?"

"Not that I remember."

"I heard you snoring."

"I was just checking on your hearing."

I did sleep through several innings of the ball game recently and there was no elbow in my ribs. Awakening, I noticed she was asleep also but I kept that to myself. I know when I'm ahead. I find I rather enjoy sleeping in the recliner but don't ever broach that feeling for fear of an argument.

She snored this morning and afternoon but she didn't hear herself. I laugh to myself. Where's the equality process?

"Go to bed if you can't keep me company," she says. This leads to stress in me. I'm feeling stress more and more often as my role as a caretaker grows.

I now write in the morning before her nortriptoline pill for migraine headaches wears off and she awakens. I have other diversions to enjoy during my waning months. Diversions are good for us. None of us know what is ahead. I'll keep busy to try to get most of my diversions finished before my life's December thirty-first arrives.

If I'd known what would happen in several weeks I'd be better prepared for the events that'll reshape both our lives. I'll miss a subtle signal that'll turn our life in another direction. Perhaps it is good that we can't see ahead. We might worry ourselves sick. Should we assemble an emergency or a crisis team? Neither my mother nor years of schooling prepared me to meet our coming calamity.

Chapter 2

Adoption and Adaptation: Who Adopted and Adapted to Whom?
Four Feet and Whiskers

Little do I know that this evening is the pause before the typhoon begins to descend upon us. The major storm that will hit us soon is just over the horizon in the next county. Batten down the hatches and watch the disturbance build as we wait.

Tonight dinner is finished and the dirty plates are at rest in the half-empty dishwasher. Turning out the kitchen light, I join JJL in the double recliner and comment, "Latte must have been waiting for you. She's not only on your lap, she's already asleep."

"She followed me to the recliner and after surveying it from the floor, made a calculated jump to land beside my legs."

"I've seen it before. You reached to pet her and she turned her head to lick your arm with her sandpapery tongue. After a few licks, I'll bet she looked at your lap and stepped onto it. In a moment she'd settled between your thighs with her head near your knees, right?"

"You're almost right. She wiggled to suggest that it would be better if I spread my legs further apart. Before long, she'll again suggest I give her more room. She doesn't even waken to send that message. Don, I forgot to get an aspirin before I sat down, would you get me one, please? I don't want to disturb Latte."

"What happened to the acetaminophen I put beside you yesterday?"

"I don't know. Mocha or I must have knocked it onto the floor. I haven't seen it all day." Mocha is our second and younger cat, JJL's idea of a gift for me.

"Why couldn't Latte have knocked it off? Is my wife showing favoritism?" I whisper to Self.

Going around the recliner, I wonder about the assignment of blame. Mocha is inquisitive and loves to play with small items. She'll probably grow out of this kitten behavior.

I find the bottle; it's been knocked to the floor and batted under the recliner. That sounds like Mocha's MO.

Latte's position in the household is something else. It is quite evident who's head of this house and chief of all personnel. Latte has been with us only thirty months. "Her rise from a house cat to the house CEO has been as spectacular as any corporate ladder-climbing in Silicon Valley," Self has murmured several times.

As I look at this beautiful Siamese queen, my mind goes back twenty years. Our oldest son, Larry, presented us with a Siamese kitten at Christmas. She was a classic beauty, regal in every way. JJL wrote Serakeet on the adoption papers in reference to Queen Serakeet of Siam. "Her everyday name will be Serri," Jacquie announced.

JJL was working at a high school library at the time, and often helped a little group of Vietnamese students. She told the kids, "We have a Siamese cat and I call her Serri after Queen Serakeet,"

When they heard of this name they became incensed. "The queen was not nice enough to have even a cat named for her. She was a bad queen!" Jacquie didn't know the queen but liked the name. It was on the adoption papers and it stayed that way.

Serri became as nice a cat as she was pretty. My dad, by then a widower, came to visit us one winter. He would tease Serri with a string, and they both enjoyed it, except when it became Serri's naptime and he was not ready to quit the game. One day he looped a string over her tail and leaned back to watch her antics. JJL was given an early dismissal and allowed to come home early that day. Grandpa heard the garage door opener as she arrived home. It was time to remove the string and avoid daughter-in-law troubles, but he couldn't catch Serri. JJL was in a good frame of mind and Dad lucked out without a reprimand. For years Dad would close his long distance telephone conversations from Kansas with, "Pull the cat's tail for me!" before he hung up.

An Old Man

He became ill and went to the hospital near his home. I talked to him in his bed the day after he was admitted. To end our conversation, I told him, "Serri hopped onto the bed last night after I crawled under the covers. She walked to my head, turned around and sat on my mouth with her tail running up beside my nose."

Dad laughed, coughed, and when he could talk again, said, "Pull her tail for me." Fifteen minutes later our son, Larry, called to say, "Grandpa just passed away."

As I lean back in the recliner my mind begins to wonder. "Dad liked animals," I said to Jacquie. "In the thirties, before I met you, we raised turkeys on the farm. As the toms began to mature and learn to strut, Dad would coach them by bending over, dropping his arms near the ground and calling, 'Stutt, stutt,' as he moved forward two or three steps, turkey fashion. He also enjoyed scratching the bull's neck and teaching a young bucket calf to butt with his head, until the calf surprised my small sister, Phyllis, by knocking her to the ground from behind. Mother ministered to the crying daughter and cancelled any further calf training without argument from Dad."

"Yes, but your dad didn't know when to stop. He carried teasing too far," my wife reminds me. The tone of her voice tells me that no further argument will be allowed on this topic. There are some things one learns quite well long before the fiftieth wedding anniversary. They must be remembered for continued happiness. It is called "give and take." One often gives and the other often takes.

"Your dad did take advantage of his first ram," JJL continues. "Your mother told me Dad bought the small flock of sheep at a farm auction, but forgot he had purchased a ram with territorial and harem-protection instincts. Mr. Male Sheep introduced himself from behind and sent Dad flying. It was then that the ornery streak in of your father reappeared."

"That ram was called Buck. Did Mom tell you about Dad walking beside the hog house when the Buck charged him at high speed? Just as Buck shut his eyes prior to impact, Dad stepped aside, and the ram crashed into the building. Another time or two of that, and the ram would avoid charging when Father was near a building. Dad pulled the same stunt with a post in a wire fence, and Buck, soon put men near fences off limits too."

"That was mean."

"Another way Dad teased Buck was to place his hands together in front and to one side. Buck would hit the item closest to him. Neither was hurt. Was that mean?" I ask.

"He should have played that way from the start."

"Here's another stunt. Dad would jump into the air and spread his legs as Buck was just ready to make contact. When Buck stopped Dad would come down astride the woolly back. Dad would also toss a car tire toward the charging ram. Buck would end up with the tire around his neck and a very sheepish look on his face."

"And your mother would say, 'Louis, you're taking advantage of that ram.'"

"He can stop charging any time he wants to," was Dad's answer. Jacquie, remember your mother living here when she couldn't live alone. She brought her dog Pirate with her. He was a Lhasa Apso wasn't he?"

"Yes," she replies, "he was not a handsome dog and he smelled. No, he stank!"

"I think Serri took advantage of him, just as Dad did the ram. Pirate had chased cats in the past but he was ordered not to chase Serri. He obeyed under your mom's managing eye. I can still see your mother getting up from her chair to go to her room, with Pirate following four feet behind. Then he would be humiliated. Serri would arrive on a dash from nowhere and bat him on the backside, walk four feet away and sit down looking the other way. He would give her a glance with his big, sorrowful eyes and continue behind Mom, his mistress."

With a smile, JJL changed the subject. "I'll always remember how Serri adopted our editors working on reports when we started our house inspection office in your art studio. She would hop onto the counter, walk on top of the four computers until she found the lady she would favor that day, lie down on that editor's warm machine and go to sleep. She appeared to be a part of the family enterprise."

When Serri was nearly eighteen, she became sick and a prescription did not help. A night or two later we took her to the all-night pet emergency room where the veterinarian gave us little hope. It was hard to say, "OK, put her to sleep."

Ten minutes later the vet returned to say, "She is no longer alive. Unless you have other plans, I will deal with the body?"

Upon awakening the next day, Jacquie said softly, "I remember how long the ride back to the house was last night. We didn't have anything to say, either of us."

"Yes. And before we went to bed, out of habit we started to check her food and water."

"The first thing to do when you get up is to clean the pans and put them out of sight in the garage."

"We didn't lose a household pet; we lost an eighteen-year-old family member. I remember checking water and food bowls routinely before I got myself straightened out."

We didn't want to get another cat right away. You can't replace a family member overnight. We had to overcome our loss.

But when we went looking for a cat, we were lucky again. Jacquie still remarks, "Don, even now, I find it hard to believe how lucky we were when we went looking for another cat. Later, I called the pet rescue group and asked, "Do you by any chance have a dark Siamese cat for adoption?"

"Yes, we do. Come out and see her. She had a bad wound on her right hip. We chanced on its healing, so we didn't put her down. It has healed, although the nickel-sized area doesn't have hair yet. It will come in soon," said the young lady vet rather proudly.

On arrival we found that this cat could pass as Serri's identical twin. We were ecstatic. The cat seemed to like us. She generously licked our hands with a wet, sandpaper-like tongue. "Oh yes," the young vet laughed, "We nicknamed her Mrs. Lickey. She licks everyone!"

The adoption was consummated when a syringe painlessly placed an identification silicon chip with our phone number painlessly under Mrs. Lickey's skin between her shoulder blades. I mistakenly thought adoption and love would cure the licking habit. I was mistaken. Licking is her way of returning love. After petting her I now provide her a bit of time to show her love to me.

Returning home, JJL said as she sat down in her recliner, "This beautiful cat was someone's nice pet before her accident." Immediately our new friend was on JJL's lap, considering herself at home. The lap, it seems, is a right, rather than a privilege. Mrs. Lickey was soon following us into the kitchen whenever we ventured that way, a habit she still pursues when it is time for food regardless of our intentions.

As a mature cat she has a mind of her own, and it appears impossible to re-program her. She will only consent to learning games and behaviors she approves. I think her software is programmed. Her default setting is learning only what she wants. In fact, she has been more successful at programming us. When in the kitchen at feeding time, she never makes any noise; she just looks up at us with her message showing in her eyes. On certain occasions I can drop onto all fours with my arms spread apart, and talk her into walking under my shoulders and stop for four or five strokes of petting. That is the only training she has allowed. Then she moves four feet away and sits down. The game is over. She will drop into the conversation pit and wait for me to swing a piece of paper along the edge for her to bat and catch, a game we co-invented.

A week after the cat came to live with us Jacquie made the first of several announcements. "First, Mrs. Lickey is a terrible name. We can't call her Serri even though this cat reminds me of her." Since she is a dark coffee brown with some toasted golden hairs, we decided to call her Latte. The second announcement came a week later: "Don, you need a cat to sit upon your lap because Latte seems to have adopted me." I wasn't quite sure about that idea, but I thought it might be nice to have a lap companion. Was this my wife's way to entice me to sit beside her more during the evenings of TV?

The next day I telephoned the agency again. "Hello, nice adoption lady. This is the Don who adopted Mrs. Lickey. Do you have another Siamese cat for adoption? Mrs. Lickey, alias Latte, needs a companion." No use advertising it was my male ego that was at risk.

"Yes, I do, but she's still a kitten. She's in a halfway house in Antioch. She'll be ready for adoption in two weeks."

"And she looks like Mrs. Lickey?"

"No. She's white with seal point markings. All Siamese kittens are white when born. She'll darken as she grows. She's a long-haired kitten."

"Call us when she's ready and we might consider her." I wasn't too happy with the idea of a longhaired cat, as I am quite bald. Could this be an ego problem? The call finally arrived, and once again we went to the little cat ranch where several dozen felines were waiting in pens for new families.

"Come in and I'll get the kitten," we were told by the lady vet.

"She's so full of life I have to keep her in the bathroom." We didn't get the full impact of that message for several hours.

She arrived with a charge at my feet as a small bundle of white fur. "She didn't stay for a visit," Self adds. She was here, there and onto everything in the room." Her hairs were reaching toward all points of a three-dimensional compass. I was surprised at the softness and amount of her fur. She had hair sticking out of her ears and downward between her toes. Her large feet were similar to those of a snowshoe rabbit. After the ladies have commented about her soft coat, they looked at me for a decision. This kitten is not what I had in mind but maybe my aged mind could change. The feeling was similar to seeing your first child in the delivery room. It was hardly "take it or leave it."

"We have a new lover," I announced with more decision in my voice than I intended. I think I, too, was surprised by the assuredness of the announcement.

"I'll put the microchip between her shoulder blades while you sign the adoption papers and the pledge that there will be no declawing," the vet says. The chip placement must have been painless, as the kitten did not flinch.

At home I told JJL, "I'll try to put my remaining doubts in my pocket. We won't worry about acceptability; she has us already! Now it's time to convince Latte that she too should adopt the tiny ball of activity. I'll be the kitten's champion."

There was a lot of hissing, spitting, wrestling and growling, which continued for several days. I swear that there was some feline cursing also! Latte's ego was wounded. She hadn't been consulted about the adoption of a younger feline or about sharing her kingdom with another.

In time JJL announced, "I think the furor has switched from jealousy and warnings to spirited play. The cats are now taking turns doing the chasing."

At night they play in the early evening and then sleep until we go to bed. Then it is playtime in the dark. We hear them playing and running into things in the dark in spite of night vision.

Once in the middle of the night Jacquie awakened me. "What's that noise in the bathroom?"

"I don't know."

"Well, get up and find out what's happening!"

It was easy to arise and turn on the light, as I was now wide-awake. I almost choked with laughter as I announced; "The kitten has found the plastic white cap that covers the bolt holding the toilet to the floor. She has pulled it off its bolt. She's intrigued by the fascinating noise and movement it makes as she bats it around on the hard surface of the floor. I'll toss it out on the carpet of the bedroom so you can get some sleep." The kitten was having a great time all by herself. On later nights, the kitten brought her beloved bolt cover to us in bed, hoping we would throw it for her to chase with a tumble and roll.

Jacquie's been in ill health for several years. Several of her prescriptions cause drowsiness. That is not a problem for Latte, who likes to sleep on a lap, but her napping habit created some surprises for JJL. Several days after the adoption, I arrived home late one morning and commented, "You're awake!"

"How can I sleep? That cat of yours won't let me." Notice the personal pronoun directed at me? I was to hear that pronoun a number of times in the near future. "She's found there is enough room to allow her to jump between my recliner and the end table. When I'm asleep she comes at dead run, jumps through that open area and lands on my stomach. This not only wakens me; it disturbs Latte's nap also. By the time I'm awake she's landed on your recliner, raced to the conversation pit and is running around inside it."

What was I to do? I moved the table closer to JJL's recliner to make the opening smaller. That meant the painkiller and the tea were closer for JJL to reach without disturbing Latte. Not all problems end up being bad.

I don't mind having some of the blame a sick person puts on a partner being shifted to the kitten, but I wonder if the kitten is unwittingly earning an unfavorable reputation as a result. I come home today to hear, "Guess what your kitten did?" There is that pronoun again, and it is my cat that is in trouble. "Also, you didn't hear it, but your cat was rolling that darn bolt cover around the bathroom again in the middle of the night."

Notice the use of the word also. The rap sheet is growing longer. "It awakened you, Jacquie?"

"You're darned right it did. Can't you glue the cap in place?"

I did glue it, but I forgot to shut the door. The glue didn't have time to set before Mocha went after it again. That is half the story. The other cap has been catnapped and now both covers are lost. It's time to clean house. On second thought, let's skip the cleaning, the caps might be found.

One day there is a painful variation of the flying leap. The kitten is already soaring through the air and headed for a lap touchdown, when JJL starts to stand up. To make the best of the emergency, the feline missile tries to make a mid-air correction with a push-off, trying to avoid a head-on crash with JJL's stomach. One paws hits that triangular patch of flesh just above a person's crotch and a toenail hooks and catches in the flesh! The young cat swung in mid air from her attached claw, and Jacquie screamed. She told me later, "I didn't have a headache at the time, so I didn't chastise the little devil." Becoming a professional lover has at last paid off for the kitten. JJL continued, "It's hard to ignore her or not like her. She hops up by my feet as I'm lying in the recliner and walks the length of me before she flops down on my left shoulder to start purring into my ear. Then those big paws start kneading my neck. That wouldn't be so bad, Don, but she is like her master. She can't sit still."

"Uh, oh," I said to myself, "the kitten is off the hook and now it's my turn. How'm I going to be charged?"

"She can't be still on my shoulder. She gets up, turns around and flops down again. Or she walks between my face and the book I'm reading with that big, fluffy tail rubbing my face." It was pronouncement time again. "Don, you should sit down and pet your kitten so she will know whose lap to sit on." I did, but the kitten feigned sleep until she found a chance to jump down and run. When she doesn't want to be held, she throws all four feet into overdrive reverse and floorboards the gas!

It was time for another JJL pronouncement; "She needs a better name than Kitten. Do you have any suggestions?"

"If she is active like I am, why not name her Dawn after me, but with a W?"

"Come off it. One Don is enough! Be serious."

"Maybe her name could relate to coffee, like your Latte's? She has a dark tail, some brown in the seal points and also on her feet."

"Keep talking."

"The whitest coffee I can think of is Mocha."

"The vet said she would darken though. What then?"

"She'll be a darker Mocha."

The name issue decided, we settled down to raise an adolescent with a fully charged battery who would liven this house of seniors. We don't have long to wait. While Latte finds a sunny spot to nap, Mocha always chooses a place where she can keep an eye on household activities. I once thought she closed her eyes. I now believe one percent of one eye is kept open as a visual alarm. Silent activity will awaken her.

It's nine-thirty in the evening and I am becoming sleepy. My pre-dawn, old man alarm clock calls me to the bathroom near four each morning and I don't get back to sleep. JJL's bedtime pain medicine still causes her to sleep late each morning. We are headed for our regular evening domestic summit confrontation. It is all familiar ground and tactics. She is not only enjoying an evening TV program, but will watch another favorite program at ten and the eleven o'clock news as well. She expects me to stay awake. To keep myself awake, I turn my mind to a story I'm writing or a painting I will start.

"Don, are you asleep?" If I answer that I'm not, I still feel put upon. She did a lot of napping today. If I don't answer, she is disappointed in me. It's a no-win situation.

"I don't think I'm asleep."

"You were snoring!"

So what, I say silently, for my ears only, and I remind myself I didn't awaken her when I found her napping several times today. I don't argue even though I was awake.

"This activity wasn't in the job description of husband, which you read before signing the marriage certificate," Self quietly reminds me. I have just learned that I'm able to snore while awake. My Grandpa Winkley used to say, "If a partner is convinced against their will, they are of the same opinion still!" This is where an aging couple begins to change behavior patterns and the nature of risk changes. The give-and-take of early marriage sometimes becomes give-and-give-again for one of the partners, not necessarily the man. One also learns that an ill spouse is not to be pushed too far. Jacquie has not felt well for several years due to headaches and allergies.

To stay awake a little longer, I'll get a drink. I'll have to get up in the night anyhow.

Arising, I am greeted with, "Now where are you going?" When

she lived with us, Jacquie's mother used to keep an eye on me whenever I got out of a chair. I remember, too, my Grandmother Winkley keeping a close eye on Grandpa Winkley. Is this lack of trust a sex-related trait that comes into fruition when women pass menopause, or do aging men need increased supervision? It might be a good question to pose to an Internet chat room but I'll not waste time researching the question. I'll celebrate that I've lived long enough to reach this stage. I'm glad I have the problem, and I'll not kill myself because of it.

"I'm going to get a drink. Do you want me to bring your medicine?"

"Yes, and another acetaminophen, please."

When I return, both cats are between Jacquie's outstretched legs. They are face to face over her knees, giving each other a facial and a shampoo. They need watching, as one may upset the other, which will result in a small scrap. A catfight between the legs is a fight to avoid at any cost. The interior sides of Jacquie's thighs carry a number of scars resulting from frightened or fighting cats.

"Here are your night pills and a glass of water." Guess what? My wife is now counting the pills, checking to see if all the required ones are present and no extra ones! She's been watching too much TV and Jessica Fletcher, the nosy lay detective in Murder She Wrote. I'm overwhelmed with her trust in me! She supervised me when I was filling the week's pillbox. But I don't take it personally as I remember that characteristic in Grandma Winkley, an aunt or two, and aging lady teachers. If it is a sex-related characteristic God created when She made humans, who am I to get upset? If God drew Her plans that way, women have an insider's advantage, I decide. I have come to accept the baggage that comes with senioritis.

"Did you take your night medicine, Don?"

"Yes." Jessica's script again, I say to myself.

"Take Latte from my lap so I can get up and get ready for bed. Careful, don't hurt her. Just put her on the chair with the pillow." I'm a kind man and I'll not hurt Latte any more than I'll hurt JJL as I help her unrobe her arthritic arms and legs. I turn back the bed covering. Once she's in bed, I medicate a toe for her. She doesn't supervise it, so maybe I'm not doing too badly. Still, I wonder why life hasn't taught me better. I'm a slow learner, I tell myself. Maybe life taught correctly and I was really asleep. JJL's in a protective mode that bothers me.

I remember a few times that I did irritate her, so maybe the tally sheet is balanced after all. I'll go to sleep hoping we both have a better day tomorrow. I'm sure that at least the cats will have another good day whether I do or not. They are a benefit to JJL's health. Her concern for them takes her mind off herself. It is not just TV all day; it's TV and cats. Latte sleeps on her lap all day and Mocha often sleeps on the top of her recliner. All three have it pretty good, whether I'm home or out delivering reports.

It's a quiet period of time before a series of events will change our lives perhaps forever. The storm clouds are just over the horizon. We have no forecast or prior warning of their presence. We'll be hit tomorrow of all days: our fifty-fourth wedding anniversary brunch at the famous Claremont Hotel overlooking San Francisco and the Golden Gate.

Chapter 3

Another HMO Adventure
JJL is MIA at the HMO

It's Wednesday already! I used to think, "Only two more days to the week-end, hallelujah!" Now in the middle years of Seniorhood I have a different attitude. It's, "There's only so many Wednesdays left in my life and today I'm using one of the few left." Tomorrow there will be one less Wednesday.

We're in the last days of June and it's quite hot. My most recent prescription is slowing my body. My mind is developing a list of things to do and how to do them, but the body is saying, "Not now, tomorrow!" I find it disturbing to not be up and busy. I turn my key, but my starter won't work; it just clicks. It's that darn medicine!

My four-way bypass surgery was four years ago, and I've felt great ever since.

My Type A behavior schema has been on track until recently. Several weeks ago I was experiencing the sensation of having a small briefcase (or a large cat) resting on my chest – the same feeling I had prior to my heart operation. After a half-day in the emergency room on the EKG machine and generous donations of blood for testing, the verdict was: "There's no problem with your heart, go see your GP." The GP refers JJL and me to a counselor who puts each of us on a pill to lessen our tensions. I think the ingredients in my pill subconsciously tell me, "Your wife may not be right, but don't argue." Her pill counsels her "You have a good mate, so don't try any more remodeling tactics." Though my pill worked, it caused side effects. I had days where I didn't care to do any physical work and could read only two or three pages of a book without a rest. I asked Doctor Banda to try me on the pill the counselor gave JJL for the same anxieties. This pill worked. I'm almost back to par, but this Wednesday is not a high-energy day. That is why I don't go out to deliver my marketing newsletter to real estate offices. But I have enough pep to plan to celebrate our fifty-fourth wedding anniversary for Sunday. I call and make reservations at the Claremont Spa and Resort Hotel in the Berkeley Hills. JJL is also not feeling well, and that is where our next adventure starts.

On Sunday, JJL awakens early so we can shower and dress. Showering takes longer now. Her balance is not dependable so we shower together. That way, I can hold her to prevent a fall. She is not strong enough to exit a tub alone or even with help so we use our large shower stall. Once she dresses, she realizes her old nemesis, diarrhea, is arriving in spite of a prescription's effort to keep it under control. After a while, she wonders if we should call and cancel our reservation. We don't, and some over the counter pills stop the problem. Dressed suitably, we head west.

We must be excited, because we arrive much too early. To kill some time, we drive into the hills above the resort. We are soon on higher, steeper hillsides where it is a wonder that architects, designers and contractors can build and anchor houses. It is as if giant swallow nests are clinging to the vertical cliffs. It is strange to see garages designed to serve as the roofs of dwellings on the downside slope sides of the roads. It must be a challenge to cut a road into these bits of cliff side. I now know why on a dry summer night, the eleven-o'clock newscaster reports that firefighters are stationed in the Berkeley hills in a preparedness mode should a fire start. These steep hills with tightly curved roads and sometimes with only one lane, must be a problem to heavy fire trucks in a hurry. What a challenge! A few years ago, the Oakland Hills Fire killed twenty-five people, and lasted for days, one of the worst urban fires in history.

The huge Claremont Spa was the home a successful California Central Valley farmer built for his wife, much as rich European men built castles for their wives. The large dining room where the Sunday brunch is served overlooks the tennis courts far below, the San Francisco Bay, the Golden Gate and San Francisco. What a view for dining! The brunch is a treat. Seafood selections include fish salads and oysters on the shell. Huge trays hold many types of cheeses. Beef and lamb are cut to request. Custom omelets and waffles tempt us to overeat early in the meal, and have no room for the other offerings. The highlight of the brunch is the desserts. There must be at least twenty-four selections. Walnut and macadamia tortes with a thick, rich chocolate coating are competing with bread pudding floating over tasty custard for the top dessert choice. Piano music entertains us as we dine. It is a grand way to celebrate our fifty-fourth anniversary.

After the brunch, as we emerge from the building into the sunshine, Jacquie says, "Don, you go get the car. I'll wait for you here." Then she stops walking and stands still. This surprises me as she has not complained about anything and the walk is downhill.

I fetch the car and help her into it. As we start to drive away, she requests, "Take a short route home, please." At home she leans back into her recliner as usual, but says; "I don't feel my best." We don't know it then, but she is leaving the October of her life. The November of her life is beginning.

Monday she has a headache and stays in the recliner all day. Tuesday she chooses to stay in bed with Latte on her lap, while on Wednesday she arises to sit in the recliner, but doesn't dress. Latte doesn't mind and is able to sleep on her mistress's nightdress quite well.

I check her temperature in mid-afternoon and it is sub normal. Her blood sugar and blood pressure are normal at five in the afternoon. But she doesn't feel well and I move to the phone to call the HMO advice nurse.

"No! Don't do that," my wife explodes with more energy than she has demonstrated all day. "She'll want me to come to the emergency room."

After I reach the HMO answering machine, I'm directed to punch in JJL's patient number and then choose from the recorded options. The clerk who finally answers listens and decides I should talk to a nurse. I am placed on another line to wait for a voice.

"Hello, I'm a nurse and my name is Martha. How may I help you?" I describe JJL's symptoms and answer Martha's questions. Martha decides to check with the advice doctor. In a few minutes she is back and tells me to bring JJL to the hospital's emergency ward, as she might be having a slight stroke or dehydration.

I dress JJL and we leave for the ER at six-thirty. She tells the cats,

"I'll be right back." She will learn later that the statement is incorrect. She will miss her promise by several days.

The ER is crowded. There are at least thirty people in the waiting room. JJL is weak, so I park her in the one chair available while I handle the registration process. The only good thing about a long wait to see the doctor is to presume the ones he calls first either have waited longer or have worse problems than you have.

Jacquie's diabetes and other symptoms must give her some priority, as she is called before one or two people who were there when we arrived. Still, our wait is over three hours.

There are three ER wards in this hospital. The A rooms contain more specialized testing systems such as EKG equipment. Jacquie is in the B room section, or Priority Two rooms, and in twenty-four hours will be in the C, or holding pen area, as we called such areas on the ranch. It is a place to wait until a hospital room becomes available. This section is to cause me concern later.

Doctors and nurses must be explicit with questions to get to the heart of a problem. A petite nurse dressed in a dull rose uniform meticulously collected JJL's vitals as blood pressure and temperature along with the first of several blood samples. In a few minutes one of the three doctors staffing this analytical post arrives with preliminary results her cumulative folder and a clipboard. His nametag said, Dr. F. J. Kins. His eyes declared his commitment to duty. He dropped his eyes to the folder to review the test results before walking to Jacquie's side. In a moment my wife commits her first faux pas. She names the day of week and the year correctly, but answers "May" as the current month, even though she remembers we had just celebrated our June wedding anniversary. The doctor makes a note and gets up to leave.

"You're dehydrated, so I'll order two containers of IV fluid. Plan on being here till early or mid-morning," the good-looking young doctor declares as he puts his pen back in his smock and leaves to see his next patient. The IV needle and tubes are put in place. We settle down to hydrating her not guessing the procedure and others to come would continue over a number of days.

"There he goes again," Jacquie says, looking through the door. I look too and see a small middle-aged man hustling towards the bathroom. What is interesting is the fact a private, uniformed security guard goes with the little fellow. Jacquie might not be feeling well but she is alert, an attribute I've noticed in a number of older ladies, particularly her mother, my mother-in-law.

The IV bottle empties slowly, and we doze frequently. JJL says, "I miss my Latte sleeping between my legs."

After five or six trips to the bathroom, spaced about ten minutes apart, the little man is transported in his bed and placed next to the ER room nerve center so the medical staff can keep an eye on him. Perhaps the room he occupied is needed. He will also be closer to the bathroom. We can keep an eye on his movements too. We notice that a nice looking young lady and an older man alternate as guards. Since the ER rooms are for data gathering, and not for entertainment, there are no TV sets in patients' rooms. The only thing to watch is the staff outside the rooms' doors.

The little sailor on his bed in front of Jacquie's door becomes our entertainment. At least we assumed he's a sailor because he's wearing a cap with a navy ship's name embroidered on it. He dozes, then awakens and sits up in bed. Even though he has four blankets he is cold. He soon has six blankets. After another nap, he searches the room with wide, awake eyes and cries loudly to everyone in general, "Somebody call the first sergeant in Martinez!" Maybe he's not a sailor. They don't have sergeants in the Navy, do they?

An ER has as many sounds as it has sights. I hear the cries of several children, including a baby. A young mother holding a crying baby has swollen eyes and is also crying. Her young husband tries to comfort her. A red-suited nurse takes the almost-new baby from its mother. She places it stomach down on her arm while she pats its back with her other hand. The baby stops crying. It is now the mother's turn to learn the procedure. She fails again, as cries soon resume. The nurse replays her magic comforting routine.

Ten minutes pass, and it is again time for the sailor to awaken. He sits up and asks, "Are my feet covered?"

"Yes," the guard says, and the patient is instantly on his back and asleep again.

The ER has a pair of doctors, several nurses and a number of student nurses with other support staff from the labs and custodial ranks to keep the nerve center functioning properly. It is a delight to observe the organization of the unit and the staff relationship with the patients.

"I don't have a car, so will somebody take me home?" our man with the covered feet asks loudly arising to an erect position. He rotates his head and looks for volunteers. Seeing none, he is instantly asleep again.

The doctor knows Jacquie is dehydrated, but he is still testing for heart problems and the possibility of a small stroke. After the first IV bottle of fluid, my wife begins a series of incidents that call the HMO staff's attention to her. The doctor asks a nurse to help Jacquie walk down the hallway a bit to see how her coordination is. As the ladies start, the doctor comes out of the room next door where he is setting a boy's broken foot. JJL then walks into the wall she is walking beside. I am pleased. When the staff observes an incident, it is more believable than when a patient or patient's spouse describes the same behavior. That behavior ends her walk and starts a second IV. She will add interesting behaviors in the next four rooms she will occupy. Those actions will be noted and observed by the staff. Hallelujah! That's part of the reason for our being here - to let the staff know what the problem is.

The third faux pas occurs an hour later as the IV bag is replaced. "Take her BP while she is lying down, and again after she gets out of bed," Dr. Lass, Dr. Kins' replacement on this later shift, tells the nurse, "and if it is OK she can go home." The first reading is within the acceptable range but then trouble starts. As JJL stands she starts to talk to the nurse.

"Don't talk or do anything," the nurse tells her. "You've ruined the test. I've got to start all over!"

This time my wife began to get dizzy, and I reached out to steady her with my arm. "You've ruined it again. Sit down on the chair behind you and I'll try a little later." The nurse and I start to help her sit but JJL all but misses the chair. It is then that the nurse says, "You're not going home this shift." After putting JJL to bed, the nurse leaves us to report to Dr. Lass who is ending his shift.

One of the new doctors is a tall, portly fellow with large, salt-and-pepper lamb-chop sideburns. I wonder how he can replace the younger fellow caring for patients in ten rooms. Then I notice that his long legs have a lengthy stride and a fast pace. His eyes seem to miss nothing as he moves about his domain. When he comes into our cubicle he says, "It's unclear as of yet what your problem is." After asking several questions, he continues, "I have asked the doctor of internal medicine who is on duty on the hospital floor to come down to check you. Meanwhile, just lie still."

My period of aching sleepiness has passed, and I waken JJL as the lady intern arrives. First there are questions and the usual stethoscope and pulse taking. "Now stick out your tongue." A quick examination of it and the lady continues, "You're still dehydrated. I'll give you some more IV when you get upstairs." She leaves and we go back to the familiar waiting mode.

The ER doctor with the lamb chop adornments finds more IV is needed and he orders it. JJL is soon asleep. At 7:55 A. M., the doctor suggests that JJL doesn't need me and that perhaps I need sleep at home. After arousing JJL enough to say, "Goodbye, see you later upstairs," I leave. I know she isn't well, but she will get the kind of monitoring she needs to assist in her improvement, if improvement is possible.

If I had known the HMO's security system breaches would rival the security breakdown in some of our nation's airports at that time, and lead to my not being able to find my wife that afternoon, I would not have left. I will become tracer-of-missing-persons for the first of several times.

Chapter 4

Our October of Life Subplots
My Three Falls but I'm Not Out!

The plot thickens. The HMO is about to dismiss JJL when they find she is not ready. They decide to keep her without placing a label on her problem. There is not even any guessing. "She's dehydrated and needs an IV" indicating a condition that needs addressing. The discovery of a more basic problem may happen.

"But why does she need IV?" Self fairly shouts at me as I exit the parking garage and head for the freeway onramp. The thirty-minute ride home from the hospital will give me time to reminisce about our pre-hospital days and see if I can answer his question.

We are into the October of our lives, and my wife is in the hospital for unknown reasons. Are we realizing this scenario as part of the fall season of life, which most seniors experience as routine? To make the remainder of our time more colorful and enjoyable, we have chosen to have pets, in our case, the cats with coffee names. The relationships we experience with them weave themselves through our autumn days like a subplot. They're good preventive medicine.

"Those cat adoptions were smart actions," Self assures me. Self's use of the word cat causes me to raise my left hand to feel the little sore bump on my forehead. My mind goes back several nights to another cat, a big one. There even was bloodshed.

One doesn't expect blood at the zoo but that is where it happened. I was at the lion cage with a grandchild. The lion backed against the loose bars of his cage, and as he did, his rear made a loose bar move. To protect my grandchild, I swung my foot horizontally, intending to land a terrific kick on his protruding parts. "Get back inside, you devil," I screamed. The lion settled into a sitting position as I kicked. I missed his lowered posterior. The force of my swing carried my foot well to the left of the lion. There was a terrific bang and I felt severe pain in my head. My foot-swing had carried me out of bed, and I found myself on my knees with my forehead against a drawer handle of my bedside dresser. I awakened instantly in our darkened bedroom.

I clasped my painful forehead and then opened my eyes to look at my hand. There is a bit of blood on it. My head hurt so much I didn't want to get off the floor! I only wanted to stay where I was for a moment.

JJL awakened, turned on a light, and all but ran around the bed to be at my side. Seeing what happened, she asked, "Shall I get an ice pack?"

"Yes."

She was back from the kitchen more quickly than she had traversed that passage in months. I was now sitting on the floor, and I placed the pack on my left temple. "It's on the other side, Don," she exclaimed, "Move it to the right!"

"It hurts here," I told her, putting my left index finger over the spot with the most pain.

"Wait a minute, I'll get my glasses." She quickly navigated around the bed to her nightstand. In a moment, with glasses in place, she assured me she was right. "Move the pack to the other side." I had lost another argument, even though I knew better. When the spot on my forehead became swollen, I would make my point, but in a silent way. It is not nice to chastise a Good Samaritan or a helpful spouse after a good deed.

How could her brain be so disoriented? Her balance problem was not present that night but the visual orientation was out of whack. Was she having a new problem? A mini stroke? Little did I know that other falls would happen to me within a week. Jacquie has told me for years that things occur in threes.

I think about my lion dream as I pass through the 680-580 interchange. Heading east, I have to face the sun climbing over the horizon directly ahead of me. Why fight it? I ask myself, and turn into the nearby IHOP. Self read my thoughts and assured me, "By the time you've finished breakfast, the sun will be covered by your visor,"

An hour later, with the pleasant taste of lingenberry pancakes still in my mouth, I arrive home to bring in the morning paper, feed the birds and cats, and take a few moments of quality time with them before falling fully dressed onto the bed. These days I'm not in the habit of staying awake nearly thirty hours at a time. I may be in my second childhood but I'm having trouble staying awake this long at a time.

I fall instantly asleep. I get to saw wood only three hours before the phone rings. As I turn to answer, Latte, who has been curled up beside me, jumps to the floor. "Hello," I say groggily, thinking the call will be from the hospital.

"Yes. I'm Jay calling from Master Card. How are you this morning?" I almost tell him, but before I can answer, he continues. "We sent you an offer for a new card three weeks ago. I'm calling to discuss it with you now that you have had time to study our offer."

"I'm not interested."

"But you will have seven thousand dollars available to you instantly, you can't beat that."

"I'm not interested."

"And you have an extra month before your first ...."

"I have too many cards now. They have caused me a physical disability."

He sounds puzzled. This isn't in his script. "What is the disability, if I may ask?"

"You may ask. Sitting on the cards has caused a dislocated bun." There is a groan and I continued, "I run a cash-and-carry operation. Goodbye!"

"Oh yes. Goodbye."

I put the phone down and lay back onto the bed. In a moment it's ringing again. I answer, "Hello." It could be the hospital. It isn't. It's another telemarketer. I engineer a shorter conversation than the previous one. Again back to the sawmill. Before I can start the saws again, the phone sounds once more. "The hospital?" I ask aloud. It isn't. A fellow artist is calling to tell me my paintings are back from a show and I can pick them up tomorrow.

Why go back to the mill and lumber now that I am fully awake? I'll call the hospital. Since JJL doesn't initiate calls, and getting a line out from her bed may be a problem, I'll call to check on her before watering her houseplants.

"Kaiser Hospital, how may I help you?"

I ask this invisible person for the room number for Jacqueline Larsen who was to be admitted this morning.

"I don't have anybody by that name registered."

"She was in the ER five hours ago. I thought she would be upstairs by now."

"I'll transfer you to the emergency department."

"This is Emergency. How may I help?"

"I am calling about Jacqueline Larsen."

"The name is Jacqueline Larsen? The name doesn't sound familiar. I'll check for you." After a short pause, "No, we don't have anybody by that name."

"She was in B 4 when I left her four or five hours ago."

"This is the A emergency area. I'll transfer you."

"Hello. This is Emergency B." After my questions, the nurse answers, "There's nobody here by that name." Jacquie has been transferred somewhere, I decide. Since she didn't have a car and hasn't been able to drive for some time, she is somewhere in the institution and it is up to me to find her. I put on a clean shirt, grab a stalk of celery to eat on the trip, and check the cat food and water before leaving for Walnut Creek. I will have to play Jessica Fletcher.

I could say it was a nice drive; however, since I will make the trip several times more before she came home, I probably should use the phrase pleasant commute. The parking lot is almost full and I use one of the few spots available. The hospital is also crowded.

"No, she's not in the hospital," I am told at the information desk.

"I'll take the matter in my own hands and locate her," I tell the receptionist as I start for the rear doors of the ER, located on the opposite side of the institution. The hospital has had several additions and appears to have turned into a maze, with corridors that don't always line up directly. Persistence pays off, and I soon arrive at B 4, but when I look into the room its male occupant doesn't look like my JJL. A nurse approaches me in what appears to be a confrontation mode. She spreads her feet spread apart in the doorway of B-4. "Where have you moved Jacqueline Larsen?" I ask.

"Never heard of that name," she announces without having to think about the question. Her hands go to her hips and her head dips to allow her to eyeball me over the tops of her glasses. "Never heard of that name!"

"She was in B 4 just six hours ago," I counter.

"You'd better go to ER admitting and ask there," she says looking me in the eye. It appears this nurse on the latest shift plans not to move until I am gone.

At the admitting desk, I say to the clerk, "Jacqueline Larsen has been moved," "Where did she go?"

After consulting the computer she answers, "C 8," and points to the hall I used to enter the B section. I am totally dependent upon a silicon chip to find my wife.

In the corridor I find the C corridor rooms numbered only to four before coming to a set of unique double doors. Like many hospital doors, they operate by push plates instead of doorknobs. Transport personnel hit the plate with an elbow as they prepare to pass through with a patient.

Back at the admitting nurse I say, "The numbers stop at the double door."

"Hit the push plate at elbow height and turn left."

I do and I find JJL at last. She is getting her fourth liter of IV fluid in a four-bed ward with curtain walls. This unit C is a holding-pen for patients waiting for a hospital bed to become available. It is a waiting place similar to purgatory, I decide. The ER staff is no longer treating her. She is waiting for the hospital group to take her social security number or name, so technically she isn't theirs yet. That will happen when they have a bed for her. She's almost fallen through the cracks.

Jacquie and I figure, incorrectly, that patients checking out by noon would leave beds available early in the afternoon. We are partly wrong. The other patients in the holding room have been there longer, and they are eligible for the first beds. Jacquie doesn't go upstairs until six thirty or seven, but what a room! It's on the third floor beside an ancient oak tree of immense proportions. She looks out her single bedroom through this huge tree to a beautiful sunset. She has a TV, a necessity for a lady who spends her days watching electronic entertainment.

The dinner hour has passed but the nurse heats a frozen meal, though not the gourmet kind I have seen Martha Stewart or Mr. Food fix. After JJL finishes eating, I say, "Goodnight, I'll see you tomorrow unless you become lost again." I don't know my smart-aleck remark will become so prophetic. I am to become proficient as a tracker of missing persons.

I couldn't know it then, but fall number two is just ahead. I should have stayed in the hospital and crawled into bed with Jacquie.

The in-house café is closed by now so I decide I will stop for an ice cream cone on the way home. It has been seven hours since my stalk of celery, and I can feel hunger pangs. I don't find parking in front of the Danville Baskin-Robbins ice cream store so I drive through the cobblestone opening to the rear parking lot. Not wanting to walk on cobblestones in the dark, I elect to use the sidewalk. It's quite dark and I don't see the edge of the sidewalk. I trip and fall landing on my ribcage on my elbow. My hands, ribcage and kneecap all call for inspection and attention. "No blood, no scrapes or breaks," I tell myself.

"Go ahead and get a dip of pistachio almond, and you'll feel better and heal quicker," Self assures me. The knee will stay dark and tender for a week. I should have put a dip of coconut pineapple on top of my first choice. I might have healed faster. The double doses would have speeded recovery I reason. As I crawl back into the car I vow to call our children when I arrive home to tell them about their mother..

The cats are the last of the family to be fed tonight. I soon go to bed, believing I know which room Jacquie will be found in tomorrow morning. I sleep well and don't find any escaping lions to kick.

Awakening, I go to the kitchen in my shorts to heat a cup of my Wake-Up-and-Go Instant. I am just reaching for the coffee container when I feel a wet, hard sanding of my left leg. Latte is asking, via her tongue, for cuts in line. She wants to be fed before the coffee is made. "It's coming," I tell her, hoping she'll understand and not nip my calf as she sometimes does after losing patience with me.

I pick up on household chores. With California's energy crises, I wash and dry clothes before dawn and tidy the kitchen. Once the wash is started, it is time for quality time with Mocha. She hops to her perch beside Grandma Hazel's old red chair where I am drinking my first cup of Wake-Up. After I pet her on one side, she turns around to present her other side. Then she drops into the chair and lies beside my leg for more petting. After the coffee and Mocha, it's a good time to do yard watering as dawn arrives. The predictions for the day indicate temperatures over a hundred degrees.

And then it happens! I can't believe it happened! Stepping up onto a terrace to add seed to a bird feeder, I don't get my foot high enough, so I trip and fall again! Fortunately, there are a lot of birdseed shells and small bits of bark on the ground so I don't hurt either my hands or my knees. It's fall #3 for me. "Things happen in threes, according to old wives' tales," Self assures me. "You're safe now for awhile." I'm not too convinced by the tone of his voice.

It's near ten as I arrive at room 3041 to find a man in Jacquie's bed, the only bed in the room. No Jacquie! At least she's not in bed with him. "How could it happen again to the same person in the same hospital? The only consistency with this hospital is its inconsistency," I complain to Self as I gear up for another lost person routine.

He lowers my blood pressure by telling me, "You can find her, Don. It's a matter of using your head. I know you can."

I tell the lady at the nursing station. "Jacquie Larsen is not in room 3041 this morning."

"No, she was moved."

"I know. That's very obvious, but where is she now?"

"Let me check." She turns to hunt for JJL on the silicon chip again. "Room 3054," the chip replies but it is the nurse who smiles.

Entering the two-bed room, I ask, "Did you get displaced from that nice room by a local political figure?"

"I don't know, Jacquie says. I just got moved. I do have a nice roommate. She just passed her driver's license at eighty-nine, and she's Portuguese. I've still got the IV. I must have been really dehydrated!"

"She looks better than she has for several months," I tell Self, and repeat it to JJL with a big grin. She often sticks her tongue out at me when receiving a compliment, and she does that today, wrinkling her nose at the same time.

"That reaction is a plus sign," Self informs me, as if I don't know.

"They still don't know what my problem is, but they keep me on the IV."

By now she needs to head for the bathroom. I have learned to unplug the IV pump and hold her arm as she heads to the little room. After returning her to the bed, I begin reading a mystery book to her. I'm becoming quite good at visiting in hospitals. I'm getting a lot of practice. I'm a professional visitor.

I open the seals on her food containers; a task she can't perform. "I imagine a great many other Octoberites suffer the same problem," I try to assure her. I then go for a snack myself. It's soon time to commute home, a thirty-minute drive. After last night's experience I don't stop for a cone of either pistachio or coconut pineapple ice cream. I have to get some things done around the house tonight. Our son and his family from Kansas will arrive in a few days.

Several days ago I ordered venetian blinds for ten small windows. They arrived yesterday by truck. I open the box of blinds, and begin sorting the packages to match to individual window frames. This draws the attention of the cats, and soon Latte is exploring inside the empty boxes while Mocha inspects the packages of blinds. Something different is always of interest to cats. After laying the blinds on the floor and removing the old hardware from window casings, I notice cat hair on the carpet. I will have to find time to brush our felines. That thought makes me suddenly tired and I decide to go to bed. As I settle under the sheet I notice Latte is preparing to sleep beside me now that JJL is not available as her bedmate.

Four o'clock seems to be an ideal time to awaken if you want to accomplish something before the day starts. I put the last load of clothes into the washer, have a cup of leaded coffee and spend quality time with Mocha. Fully alert now, I heed the blinds as they call, "Get us up before you bring JJL home." As I finish the drill and template work, I hear the weather person on the TV forecast temperatures of a hundred or more for our area again, so I stop being a blind man and become a gardener as I water our vegetables and flowers.

Back inside I call Jacquie. "Hello. How are you doing?"

"Not good! I had a very bad night. Come right over and I'll tell you what happened. I need you!"

"I hope you didn't switch rooms again. I'll shave, dress and be right over."

"Make sure the cats have food and water, Don."

As if I didn't have enough worries my constant companion Self whispers in my ear, "They've changed rooms on you in short order in the past Don. 'Wanna take any bets this time? You've got a losing streak going, so what say?"

Chapter 5

Fiasco at the Doctors' Office
Where Did the 12 IVs Go?

"What can Jacquie's problem be?" I ask Self. "For years I've believed she's attracted problems. I hope its only hand-holding she needs this morning, but she did sound almost frightened."

After changing from gardening clothes, I turn to make the bed. Mocha sees me pick up one corner of a sheet and realizes it is bed-making time. She leaves the dining room at full tilt, takes to the air five feet from the bed and almost jumps over it. She loves bed making. She rolls, pats the bed clothing with her paws and emits little kitten-like sounds. To speed my sheet arranging I toss her to the floor, but this only results in another jump to where the action is, with more rolling and tumbling. I throw the sheets to the head of the bed and she is covered. That seems to be OK by the rules she uses. I pet Latte, who is sunning herself on the rug in my studio, and then I'm off to see what JJL's statement, "I need you," is about.

As I reach for the garage door I see Latte by the cat's water bowl. She looks up at me as if to say, "Fill the bowl, please. Who knows how long you'll be gone." Like her mistress, she is the master of silent communication. All it takes is for our eyes to meet. I wonder if all cats have that ability, or if it is a trait of the females, regardless of species. Another theory crosses my mind. Since dogs are reported to look like their masters, maybe cats can act like their mistresses. I wonder if I could get some federal grant money to pursue such an investigation. With the Internet I could raise a cadre of retired assistants. In fact, there may be enough right here in Livermore, home of a national laboratory whose main work is research. Maybe I have the process backwards. Maybe I should contact some retired lab workers first, as some of them have spent half a lifetime obtaining research money for much less interesting activities.

Even though it's Saturday, the last day of June, the pre-July fourth holiday traffic is moving rather well and I'm soon in the hospital parking garage. Two nights ago, I forgot which floor I was parked on and had to check several floors before I found our car. The south garage has five levels, each with four rows of twenty-five cars per row. I've seldom used the north unit, which has an equal number of spaces. Since the levels are color-coded, I'll see if remembering a color is easier than numbers for my stumbling memory. I find a spot on the floor with red support posts. I'll remember that as the ketchup floor. Yesterday I parked on the mustard floor.

Although I laugh about my forgetfulness, I do have a legitimate problem. Like thirty-per-cent of those who under go heart by pass surgery, I lost some memory. When the breathing and blood circulation is transferred to and from the refrigerator-sized machine the brain may not receive its full complement of oxygen and a few brain cells die. Brain and nerve cells don't regenerate like muscle and skin cells. The operation took me from a lethargic person to an active one. This is better than the alternative, a perfect memory six feet down.

I find myself behind a geriatric driver who wants the first parking space available on a lower floor. She stops to wait for a person returning to a car, only to find the person has came back for a forgotten purse or magazine. By the time the false lead dawns on her, the lady has four other cars stopped behind her. I'm not so picky about where I park. I've found it takes no longer to walk to the elevator on the fourth or fifth floor than it does on the second.

I again wonder if JJL is going to be in the same room I left her in yesterday. I feel positive and punch the #3 button of the hospital's elevator. While I have a slight worry about what I will find, I meet hallway and elevator occupants with a smile or a thumbs-up gesture. I am rewarded with smiles. A hospital should be as happy a place as possible. I've always believed we create much of our luck and mood, and I thrive on my casual relationships. I also believe my upbeat countenance helps others even if only for a moment. Perhaps it is my odd looks or an unbuttoned shirt or fly that draws the smile. I did forget to pull my zipper up several days ago. I hope I don't get like many older fellows and forget to zip it down.

I enter room 3054 and it's my Jacquie in the bed with tubes running into her. She throws me an unusually bright smile. She is not a demonstrative or enthusiastic person, but I beam a big smile at her as I hurry to her bedside. Our hug feels good to both of us. One benefit of the October of life is giving and receiving one more hug. At this stage of life one never knows when the benefit will be curtailed or recalled. At any stage, really -the disaster at the World Trade Center brought that concept home.

Speaking of hugs, I remember one of JJL's wardmates in the ER holding area several days ago. He was an old fellow, finishing his November years and checking into December. Spousal hugs weren't to be a part of his healing process for awhile. Preparing to admit him to a hospital room, the nurse asked for nearest of kin. "Do you have a wife?"

"Yes."

"She lives at the same address?"

"Yes."

"We can get in touch with her at the same phone number?"

"No, she's in the hospital here somewhere."

I am glad JJL and I take turns being ill. We usually rise to the need to help the other at such times.

"Now, what happened last night?" I ask.

"I fell out of bed in the middle of the night."

"You were kicking lions?"

"No. I had to go to the bathroom and I hurried too quickly."

"Did the nurse lose hold of you?"

"I wasn't quite awake, and I forgot to call her. I got dizzy, and as I fell I tore the IV needle from the back of my hand."

"Did you get to the little room in time?"

"I don't want to talk about that. I'm so glad you're here. Give me another kiss and just hold me a minute. I awakened the nice lady next to me, and she called the nurse, bless her."

My presence seems to be good medicine as JJL settles back against her pillow with more contentment than I've seen since she was admitted. I had a new mystery book to read to her, but she is watching the Masters golf tournament. She was never an athlete, nor did she enjoy sports, but in the last decade of her September years, she developed a sports interest by default. Now in what may be her November years she has the TV on a lot, and finds sports more enjoyable than the soaps or reruns. I put the book down and settle back to make the most of the event. I enjoy the staging and announcing and her interest in the players. She recognizes them and calls their names.

When the game ends, I reach for the book. "Oh good," she exclaims, "Wimbledon is going to be shown next." I lay the book down and prepare for a lesson about tennis. It is great to see her in such good spirits. Last week at home, she wasn't watching TV. She was only listening with her eyes shut. This is much better. There is hope now.

"It's Hallelujah time again!" Self almost shouts.

I look up later and see Mrs. Wall and several other women going into the Family Room across from Jacquie's domain. Mrs. Wall drove Dick, her husband, to the last session of my Tuesday writing class. He has terminal cancer, and I learned last week that he has only days left. I meet her eyes as she leaves the family room. She recognizes me and steps to our door. "Dick is just down the hall. He had a bad night."

Three hours later, she again appears at the door to say she needs some caffeine and asks, "Mr. Larsen, would you join me for a soda?" As we relax on the shaded patio by the hospital cafeteria, she asks, "Did you know Dick didn't work those word search puzzles you gave him at class? He brought them home to me and I enjoyed them."

Self whispers to me, "Bring her a handful tomorrow. Perhaps she needs something to help pass the time, as TV is not part of Dick's December thirty-first vigil."

Dick had been writing his autobiography, and has only completed it up to their marriage. When he could no longer write, the family gave him a voice-operated tape recorder. Mrs. Wall and Dick's brother Jim will try to finish the work later.

A nurse takes JJL's oxygen away. She's now free to walk while pushing a battery-powered IV pump tower. We go for a stroll and she is surprised to hear me call out, "Hi Virgil!" And to Jacquie I say, "You remember Julie, who taught third grade for me, this is her husband." She nods, and I ask Virgil why he is here.

"Julie fell and broke her thigh bone at the socket ball, two weeks after she got home from her operation for a brain tumor," he tells us.

An Old Man

"She's coming through this OK, though."

I look in the room and say, "Hi, Julie." If principals are allowed to have favorite teachers, Julie was one of mine. JJL and I finish our walk

Jacquie is doing better. She urges me to go home and get some rest. I take her advice, not to rest but to go home. I do some work on the blind installation; I want her to be surprised when she gets home. Then I hit the sack, as I am tired. I'll finish in the morning when I'll be more alert.

It's a great morning. At my age any morning is a great morning! Shortly after five I have my quality time with Mocha and a cup of coffee. My day is off to a great start already! I soon finish the last stage of window blind installation. Jacquie will be pleased with the new blinds, I hope. That is my rewarding thought. Since it reached 109 degrees in Livermore yesterday, the hottest place in California, I decide I should do another watering routine now that dawn is lighting the yard. While the exterior plants are getting their morning moisture, I water her indoor plants. The next chore is to empty the dishwasher and reload it. I will tell her to stay in the hospital, as I don't want her home messing up my clean house.

"You'll get the wrinkled nose and tongue routine if you tell her that," Self assures me.

"All the more reason to say it."

With household and yard chores complete, it's time to shower and dress for visitation. On the way to the freeway I stop to present Rosie, my eighty-five year-old neighbor, with some more turnips. Many would laugh at this gift, but she likes my excess roots. I believe elderly ladies like to have a visitor bearing gifts now and then. "Thank you, I'll have more stew," she exclaims.

Then it's Freeways 580, 680 and the Main Street turnoff. It's Sunday, so many of the hospital offices are closed and I'm able to park on the third, or Mustard, level. "I hope she didn't fall out of bed last night," Self whispers in my ear.

"When I called to say I was coming she sounded fine," I retort.

She's in good spirits. The curtain between the two beds is drawn back, so I greet her roommate, "You're looking well."

"I am, and your wife had a good night. She didn't fall out of bed and we've been visiting all morning." I can't remember when Jacquie has visited with anyone other than family. This hospital stay is having some great side effects.

The golf tournament is on again, and after a hug and kiss, I settle down to help watch it. I can entertain myself, as I am a doer more than a watcher, but sharing her activity will help me develop the next hours into quality time for JJL and myself.

We have just settled into a comfortable mode when a visitor walks into the room. "Hi Grandma." It's Melani, a granddaughter who works in Colorado Springs. I noticed the TV is immediately turned OFF. I didn't command that much response when I walked in.

Mel, her nickname, is our daughter Karen's oldest. It appeared this child would never mature. She enjoyed college and finally joined the Air Force. Maturity evolved in a hurry. Fortunately, she retained her delightful vigor and enjoyment of life while becoming a responsible young adult. She trained in the computer fields and with her military clearances soon found work in the civilian world upon discharge. .

Our blond Melani is an accomplished visitor at the master degree level. She immediately settles into an easy-relating mode and time begins to pass more quickly. Jacquie is enjoying herself more than she has for many months. "This is another great side effect," I say to Self. When Mel's remarks about how well Grandmother looks, I chip in with my own comment, "I agree Mel. I think she should stay here awhile longer. This place seems to agree with her." This causes my wife to stick out her tongue at me, much to Mel's delight.

Mel gets her own tonguing and wrinkled nose when she chirps, "You're right, Grandpa!" Then she asks, "What do they think is wrong, Grandma?"

"I was terribly dehydrated, and that's the reason for the many bags of IV they're giving me." A later count comes to twelve bags of this fluid of life. "I also apparently had a light stroke or two." We go on to tell how she had mis-functioned a time or two recently. "And perhaps I had a mini-stroke awhile back. Don said I had slurred speech one night."

"It was all run together," I say. "When I said, Huh, she accused me of not wearing my hearing aids. She wouldn't repeat herself and went to bed. I now think it was slurred speech rather than me not listening. This might have been one of her first strokes."

"By the way, when's Larry getting here?" Mel asks us.

"They were to leave last Friday," I reply.

"I want to see them, so I think I'll have a barbecue at my folks' ranch Sunday and have them up."

Time has flown and Mel is getting ready to go back to her parents' ranch. Since they picnicked mid-afternoon, she plans to stop somewhere for a snack.

Looking at me, Jacquie suggests, "Why don't you go along with Mel? You and she can eat together somewhere. The snack bar downstairs has closed by now."

I take her suggestion and Mel and I enjoy a meal together at a pancake restaurant. "At one time, she worked for our house inspection company. It was a delight to visit about what she had done since helping me market our inspection firm to Realtors. We did a lot of remembering as we ate. She is a consultant and sales person so the experience of walking into Realty offices for us years ago was good training. "Even in those early years, she was at ease meeting strangers," Self whispers to me.

I reply, "I don't think she ever met a stranger." To Mel I state as I pay our bill, "Grandma enjoyed seeing you and she'll look forward to the picnic."

When I arrive at home, I get cola from the frig and head for the red platform rocker. I barely settle into it when Mocha arrives with a flying leap on the feline penthouse roof next to the rocker, inviting me to pet her. She is excited as she climbs up and down from this perch, and knocks over my cola. I vow never to place a drink near the perch in the future. It is obvious that she is lonesome and needs immediate attention.

The next morning I treat myself to an outdoor breakfast at sunrise. I enjoy the treat, as my wife would rather not be outside at this stage of her life. As I finish with a large mug of coffee, I am careful to be quiet, and I'm rewarded with the sight of a number of the birds I try to attract with feeders. The hummingbirds are the first to arrive. They come within a few feet to study me from several angles before going to their feeding. A pair of brazen blue jays comes to the feeder to quickly snatch several of the shelled peanuts I have put out for them. One of the rules in the bird kingdom, it seems, is, don't go near when a blue jay is feeding. The little yellow-breasted finches are soon feeding, too, as they hang upside down and sideways on the bag of thistle seed hung from the birch tree.

It's time to go inside and tidy the house before leaving for the hospital. As a change from my wife's usual TV sound, I'm cleaning to semi-classical music.

It's a typical morning at the hospital until Jacquie's doctor arrives. "You were very badly dehydrated. You must drink eight glasses of water a day," he says, as he shakes his finger at my wife. "I think you had a slight stroke or two," and he goes on to define the condition. "I don't know about your heart yet. We've monitored it, but I am considering a stress test. First I need to know if you are willing to undergo two other procedures if the stress test suggests them."

"I can't do the treadmill test, Doctor."

"No, no, I will inject some chemicals into the blood to get the same results."

"That's no problem."

"But I need to know if you want to go ahead with an angiogram and perhaps bypass surgery if the stress test merits those procedures. There is no need to do the test if you won't say yes to a follow up procedure if it is needed."

"I don't know," Jacquie says and looks at me. I shrug my shoulders and suggest another fifteen or thirty years with me might be just what she needs. She tells the doctor, "Yes. Don has had both and I need to keep up with him."

""I've not seen her so positive lately," Self gasps. In a moment he continues, "Don, you'd better get three wishes ready."

"Such as?"

"First she does the test and there is no need to thread the little camera up a groin artery to the heart."

"And I suppose the second is, if they must search, hope the artery doesn't have any blockage needing a reopening or a by pass operation? What's the third?"

"Hope that if there is blockage it can be treated by placing a tiny metal tube, called a stint in the artery by inserting it through the artery rather than the more major operation, a by pass."

The doctor interrupts our conversation. "Then we will do the test first thing in the morning. We'll withhold dinner tonight." The doctor smiles and leaves for the next patient. We don't know then that she will shake up the medical staff fifteen hours later as they begin the procedure. She is still full of surprises. What a wife!

An hour later, a gurney driver comes for her. We go through the maze where the older and new buildings join at odd junctures, to finally arrive at the lower-level ICU center. She is settled into a bed, and will spend the night there before the stress test. Another room, I note. Self whispers with a giggle, "I hope you find her here tomorrow when you arrive."

At home again, I am greeted by the cats who are waiting inside the door with upturned eyes. Again, the silent language. They heard the big garage door open and close, and know dinner will soon be ready.

As I return the cat food container to the refrigerator, the phone rings. "Hi Dad." It's Larry, our oldest son. "We're in Berkeley at Karen's parents' place. How are you and how's Mom?"

"She's in Kaiser's ICU at Walnut Creek and they're trying to find out how she is." Larry is a paramedic in Wichita and his wife, Karen, is a nurse in the Trauma Center there. He is brought up to date, and we exchange phone numbers, including those of our cell phones, for use tomorrow.

After finishing the call, I replace the receiver and to collect the mail. Larry is on my mind. It will be good to see him and his presence will do his mother a lot of good. Reading my thoughts, Self agrees, "Yeah, he'll be better for her than three acetaminophen, a nurse and you, Don. You'll have to admit, he was an interesting one to raise."

"You got that right. He needed a strong set of reins and a halter that had visors limiting his side vision. He steered better going down a lane than across an open field."

"What set him apart from his older sister, Karen, was that she learned by seeing others make a mistake. He didn't. In fact, if he failed, he'd back off and charge the same problem again."

"He enjoyed his high school sports, Don. Wrestling, football on a muddy field and soccer were his life. I think your being a vice-principal and knowing the local policemen helped him make better decisions than several of his friends."

"Yeah, and working a night shift at a filling station helped also. He came home tired and ready for bed. Self, do you remember the night JJL and I brought home a white box of food from a Chinese meal?"

"Fill me in."

"We put the leftovers in the box and as the fish was served as a whole unit, we broke off the head and put it on top before closing the lid. We went to bed but Larry went to the refrigerator for food when he came home. He opened the box to be greeted with a fish head with open eyes looking up at him. He lost his appetite and was soon in bed."

After graduation he joined the Air Force and served in Viet Nam. Upon returning and marrying he plastered pools and became a partner in a termite company. As Grandpa Larsen began thinking of retiring from the family farm, Larry moved to Kansas with Susie, his first wife, and girls Kriss and Becky. Becky's kitten wakened her one night as the house was catching fire. They escaped with their nightclothes. JJL and I went back at mid winter break and helped them with a modular house. It was the weekend of the first Super bowl.

Later they left the farm and started a business in Peabody. One of his buildings had an apartment and as my mother had passed on, Larry installed his grandpa in it near the business.

"Don, Larry and his grandpa were very close weren't they?"

"Yes. Do you remember when JJL and I went to see my folks when he was a baby? Larry would fuss and cry. My mother, a proud lady, would take him from Jacquie to quiet him to no effect. Dad would come near and Larry would twist in her arms and reach to his grandpa. Once in Dad's arms the crying stopped. Neither Mother or Dad could completely hide their feelings.

After separating from Susie, he met another Karen while training to be an EMT. They married and we have two Karens in the family They have two little boys, Lucas and Keifer. Karen works in a trauma unit of a Wichita hospital and Larry runs an ambulance. Off shift and on weekends, they man the EMT unit in Peabody.

The next morning I find my way through the maze of halls and floors to the ICU rooms. After checking on Jacquie, I go to see her former roommate, thinking she would like a report. The report is interesting. The roommate tells me my wife stirred up the staff again. Instead of falling out of bed, she up chucked at the stress test. This had never happened before, and most of the staff dashed to the scene to help. "How could you do this on an empty stomach? We withheld your breakfast!" the doctor asked. One of Jacquie's problems is a valve on the lower end of her stomach that diabetes sometimes affects. The valve doesn't open to drain the stomach when it should, hence her habit of vomiting at odd times. My quiet spouse is still displaying untypical behavior that is sure to keep medical attention focused upon her.

I tell her, "It is time for another Hallelujah! The more odd behavior, the more attention you receive. And the extra attention you receive should work to eliminate your problems." She reluctantly agrees with me. Her shyness seems to disappear when surrounded by this caring staff. We have heard of uncaring HMOs. This Kaiser staff is an exception. They are great.

A few minutes later, Larry and the doctor arrive in her room at the same time. "She doesn't have a heart problem," the doctor states, and gives her prescriptions and directions.

She is dismissed in late afternoon. I am to make an appointment later in the week with her resident internist, which turns out to be another mini disaster. We pack her few belongings and another set of hospital socks, and head for home. You know you have had problems when you have more hospital socks than ordinary ones.

"The blinds look great, Don!" she says upon seeing them. Latte gives her the typical warm greeting as she wet-sands her mistress's hand. Typically she is standoffish for the next day or two. Serri, an earlier Siamese cat, behaved the same way after being left alone.

JJL takes her evening medicine including one of the large brown and tan capsules the hospital doctor prescribed. A few minutes later she develops an intense headache. The doctor had warned she could no longer take any aspirin derivatives while on this gargantuan pill. We have another problem,

I call the advice nurse, and rate the pain as fifteen on a one-to-ten scale. After consulting a drug encyclopedia, the nurse says, "That drug causes bad headaches." We find a prescription Jacquie has in the cabinet that is compatible. My wife takes it and is soon asleep.

The next morning she feels fine, but doesn't want to use the walker, which the doctor ordered her to use from now on. I bring her the newspaper, and as she reads, I pet Mocha with the petting glove I purchased recently. It's designed to remove any shedding or loose hair like cat combs. My pet tries to play with the glove. It becomes a game for a few minutes until she realizes she enjoys the petting. I soon have a glove covered with white hair. If only JJL was still spinning wool. She could create an interesting and a very soft item. Mocha is purring in a very lady like manner. Her eyes are closed and we are both happy.

Not only are we at home, we are able to go to our son-in-law's ranch for the family gathering for the Fourth of July. We are happy.

Then comes Friday. Jacquie has an eleven-thirty appointment with our family doctor. This is the hospital follow-up, and things disintegrate rapidly. "Hang on, here we go again!" I realize as I take her into the medical facility. "What's next?"

She's weak, so I put her into a wheelchair for transport upstairs to the doctor's office. She feels too sick to go on, but her streak of being at her worst in front of nurses and doctors is continuing. Great! The nurse cannot get her blood pressure. The doctor orders an IV so there will be something to measure. Where did the twelve units go? "What's happening to me," Jacquie asks, but without feeling.

I take my wheel-chaired wife to the diabetic nurse for instructions on needlework with insulin. Jacquie is feeling very ill, but the problem only gets worse.

The nurse cannot find a blood vessel for an IV needle. Jacquie's arm is yellow, black and dark rose from past needles and falls. We return from the diabetic nurse's office to the doctor who finally locates an artery with her stethoscope. Soon the IV is flowing. My diabetic is hungry, so she drinks the liquid diet the nurse gives her. It's four-thirty when our little appointment finally ends.

By the time we get home, Jacquie is feeling much better. Latte is at the door to greet her, and that is perhaps better than a kiss from me. She puts on the new housecoat I bought her recently and all appears to be well again.

Almost before she eased into her recliner, Latte is on her lap, positioning herself into one of her favorite napping locations. A moment later Mocha arrives and settles on the wide top of JJL's chair to stake out her nap site. Whether my wife feels better or not, she knows she is loved, an important medication to any ill person.

It looks as if Jacquie's health has stabilized and things are settling down to normal —or are they? Time will tell. The only thing predictable about Jacquie's health is its unpredictability.

Chapter 6

My Second Sweetheart
Programmed by the Cats

My wakeup call comes at four thirteen this morning. It is apparent Mocha has visited my side of the bed during the night. Her favorite toy, a red knitted yarn bell with a brass tinkling bell inside it, is on my side of the bed. While the coffee heats, I dress against the chill of the cold house.

I wonder where Mocha is as I head for my early morning coffee chair, the old red rotatable platform rocker Jacquie despises. This is a plain and well-used piece of furniture, but Mocha claims it as her own. She flies through the air to land on top of it, then stretches out on her stomach, with all four legs dangling down. Often the force of her landing will rotate the chair several inches. From this vantage position, she can nap or observe what's happening in most of the house's open interior. This morning she comes from somewhere at a fast pace beats me to the chair. She brings the red bell she borrowed from the Christmas tree several months ago. It's a daily toy. After dropping her toy at my feet, she utters a soft greeting and rubs against the rocker, her signal that she is ready to receive petting or retrieve the bell if I will throw it. "She's my cat," I think. "We have our routine down pat."

"Watch it or she'll have you programmed," Self giggles in my ear.

Finishing the coffee and petting means it is time to go to the computer. Mocha runs across JJL's desk and onto mine before I can seat myself. There is another soft feline "Hello" as she snuggles against my mouse hand. In time she is content to settle on her towel beside my keyboard and go to sleep. At last I have the keyboard to myself..

Looking over my left shoulder, I think I see the morning star. It soon disappears behind a mullion of my glassed studio wall. It is a pre-dawn plane headed for San Francisco or Oakland. Soon it will be light enough to do the three-mile round trip walk to Safeway's bakery for a breakfast roll. Like many other seniors, we have learned to watch our calories. JJL's diabetes demands that she be careful of sugars. Eight grams of sugar per serving is her limit. The almond roll I bring back from these early morning trips has no frosting, and half of one does not put her into sugar danger. This is a great motivation for me to do my walking. The walk for the roll has become a routine activity.

Mocha, curled into a ball, remains asleep on her towel. A rear leg passes in front of her head and the foot extends beyond her ears. My writing can proceed uninterrupted, or so I mistakenly think! I start proofing yesterday's work and open the center desk drawer for a red pen. Mocha may be asleep, but her hearing is still turned to the stay alert mode. She rises to inspect the pen, then stretches out across my notes. The angelic smile on her mouth verifies my assumption that she is a happy cat.

I'll use Mocha as the subject for my piece of class-work. The class is all seniors. Seniors like cats, and the reverse is also true, I believe. "What will I use for a title?" I ask myself.

Our Angelic Devil

A little white furry ball of Heaven arrived to live with us several months ago. She is, we think, a Siamese kitten and perhaps a very distant relative of our older resident Siamese, Latte.

A book about cats suggests we are wrong. It informs us that we probably have a Birman, an offshoot of the Siamese. The book's description and our kitten's characteristics are identical!

While many Siamese kittens are white at birth and have dark ears, tails and nose like this one, Mocha has other characteristics that are Birman like. Instead vertical eye pupils, our kitten has large, round pupils, which often appear to be dark red. The long white hairs growing outward and downward between the toes of her snowshoe-sized paws catch our notice, as do the large number of long hairs extending from inside her ears. Her whiskers are exceedingly long. Any description under her mug shot on a "wanted" poster must state that her long hair is very fine and soft, with blending blotches of lavender-tan. Her tail hair is long, dark and arranged in the style of a bottlebrush. Like the rest of her body, this bushy appendage is fascinating. It has hairs that are clear or colorless like fiberglass, and which extend beyond their darker relatives. These long strands can be seen only when she walks through sunlight, which makes them glisten like lit fiberglass strands. Another discriminating habit on her MO is carrying her tail in an erect manner, or curled toward the neck and ears.

Kittens are by nature quite active. Mocha goes beyond that. Her hyperactive behavior suggests that perhaps Heaven is not her point of origin after all. She never walks; she sprints. She will run to a thrown plaything, fall upon it and roll over a time or two before bringing it back for another try. We have considered asking her to "Fetch," a dog retrieval term. She has learned to access chairs, nightstands and anything within jumping reach. Loose pencils and pens are knocked to the floor to be batted around the room. Then it is the hearing aids that turn up missing. She once managed to remove the toilet bowl bolt-covering caps, and when she bats them about the hard floor it makes an unusual and frightening sound in the middle of one night.

Mocha's attitude is as positive as her actions. Her purring device is stuck in the ON position, although the audio output is not great. When we want to pick her up to pet her, she agrees, but only for a moment. Then all four paws shift into instant reverse, she pops her clutch and she is gone. However, longer petting sessions are beginning to become more acceptable to her.

The book states the Birman is a "People's Cat." The breed wants to be around people, and individual cats can be great companions. Mocha not only naps near us but she follows us about the house like a puppy. She can be asleep and yet hear us walk sock-footed across the carpet.

She goes to the kitchen where she earns a straight A in vocal begging. At first we thought she would turn into a glutton. Now it appears her presence in the kitchen may be as much a sign of curiosity as hunger. She wants to check everything, but is becoming less interested in eating strange things.

She does a happy purr when lying on my reclining wife's shoulder and kneading her neck with those huge paws. It becomes a problem as Mocha continually tries to find a different position. "She is like her master. She can't stay still." my wife complains. At my age, I take that as a compliment. Sleeping on the recliner back above our heads is one of her favorite pastimes.

Bed making is great fun for her as she jumps onto or under the sheets or pillows. Since she follows us, she is always there at sheet-changing time. The same is true when we change footwear. She walks beside or between our feet with a rub and a purring sound. My interpretation of that purr is, love, love, and love. A few months ago, JJL's shoe strings were a magnet to draw her. Flopping onto a newspaper I'm reading on the floor or onto clothing laid out for dressing is habitual behavior of hers.

Jacquie is never alone in the bathroom. Both cats awaken from naps to accompany her in a follow-the-leader parade of two females. As the cat book states, a Birman is a People Cat.

I set up a village of open cardboard boxes and a brown grocery bag for the cats in the living room. Hiding in a grocery bag or box is as much fun as if it were a hundred-dollar pet house. Latte was sitting in front of the grocery bag yesterday when Mocha dropped upon it from their perch above. The collapsing bag made a terrific noise. Almost asleep, Latte jumped eighteen inches into the air with her hind feet coming down almost in front of her front feet.

The only time Mocha wasn't a people's cat is when I called 911. The flashing red light and noise of the big fire truck before dawn had her total attention. When the firemen in large yellow coats came through the front door, Mocha streaked under the bed. As I left on the ambulance gurney a few minutes later, she was still there, peering from under the bedcovers.

Later, when I read the piece at class I note smiles and occasional heads nodding. They have had similar experiences with a cat. Self agrees, "Whether your teacher liked it or not, Don, these elderly ladies enjoyed it. You did it up right."

When I finish my writing, it is time for my walk. Yesterday I walked over the crest of the railroad overpass with no tiredness from the climb. It was downhill as I continued the second half of my trip to Safeway for a breakfast roll. The sun just climbing over the Altamont Pass lighted the brilliant breasts of several meadowlarks heading for their breakfasts in an open field. In the overcast, rainy afternoon predicted in a few hours, the larks' waistcoats would have little or no color.

On my walk today, I find I am walking quite fast, not only on the level, but also up the overpass. No problem, I think. However, it does take longer for me to recuperate from the walk once I am home. In fact, I have no desire to do anything until mid-afternoon. Then I decide to install our new phone.

I wonder, "Is my decreased hearing due to all the unsolicited calls I answer?" I had agreed to accept a digital phone offer, and the hardware installation is scheduled this morning. "What is a digital phone, and what does it do for me?" I ask the installer.

"Well it....." he starts. When he finishes I know little more than before asking the question. I am not familiar with the jargon he uses. I need a digital dictionary or a jargon handbook. I determine he knows more about the installation than he does about lay explanations of this technical subject. He can't talk in ordinary language.

He leaves me an additional phone I can plug into an inside jack. I decide to put it near JJL's side of the bed, so I need to install another outlet. With a new cord for under the house and a jack, I set to work. Both cats suspect something afoot and come to supervise or rather "snoopervise." Before emptying the lower part of the closet and lifting the crawlspace trapdoor, I put the cats and their portable latrine into the spare bedroom.

You never want a cat in the crawlspace. I learned that early in our house inspection business, which our son, Jon, now operates. A cat can outrun a crawling person paws down. I had a Realtor try to help me remove a cat from a crawlspace by bending into the crawl hole to grab the animal. Her action only scared the cat into running in another direction. With the Realtor lady away from the access, I succeeded in the cat eviction at last after crawling to wherever it ran several times and trying to drive it towards the opening. .

Replacing the hatch and replacing the closet items after the installation, I let the cats out and announce to Jacquie, "I have a dial tone, the cats are out of their holding room and I'm going to leave the placing of mounting screws wait until tomorrow. I'm bushed and I don't want any supper." I have a cup of strong coffee, hoping to get some snap. After lying on the bed for awhile I give up.

"You said you were going to run right up to death's door; no slowing down for you," Self laughs into my ear.

I replied, "If I can't do that, and if this afternoon's lack of energy is to be my role in my final years, it will be purgatory before death rather than afterwards."

Lying on the bed with my eyes closed, I remember one memorable crawl space two decades ago. As I approached the house with first-time buyers, I said, "This house will have an interesting crawl space."

"Why do you say that?"

"See the torn crawlspace screen vents just above the ground and along the side of the house. That first one has a large hole in the screen, and I see cat or other animal hair on the screen." The last part of a house inspection occurs in the area under the house. I pull up the hatch located in the entry closet in this mode. The odor of cats or their toilet is overpowering. This area probably serves as the cat latrine for the entire neighborhood. It is a place where they can be safe from stray dogs when they didn't want to be surprised or disturbed.

The husband and I put on crawl suits and go below to explore and inspect. I develop a headache before I have gone many feet into the area. There isn't a smell; there is a stench! After completing the crawl around the area on our elbows and stomachs, we stand in the hatch opening as we drop our suits around our ankles. Then we sit on the floor and turn the suits inside out and withdraw our feet so as not to drop dirt onto the floor of the house. I throw the suits into the truck and come home.

Entering the house in my street clothes, I take only a step or two before a finger points me back to the garage with an admonition, "Strip to the birthday suit and head for the bath tub." I do. I pull my belt and throw it into the house to use with the clean trousers I will wear. Serri, our cat at the time, came to smell the belt. She lays on it and pushes herself the length of it before flopping on her other side to slide the belt's length again. She has found hidden messages, and they are loaded with descriptions.

But back to last evening. On top of our bed, I watch a seven-thirty TV program. Jacquie catches me asleep and puts me under the covers. I let her do this thinking I feel worse than she does. Since her balance and dizziness is increasing, I usually dress and undress her. In fact, the doctor tells her to not bend over. She is to undress herself I believe by sitting on the bed. I go to sleep remembering one night I put her to bed and received a surprise reprimand during the process.

An Old Man

I guess I asked for what I got.

Her health has deteriorated for several years. One of her problems is keeping her balance while standing. At bedtime, she checks to see that I did turn off the TV, lock the doors, take my bedtime pills and turn down the thermostat as I lead her to the bedroom. That night she was wearing only a day coat with snaps down the front. Her hands do not have the strength to open snaps so I grab the two sides of the top of the coat and throw my arms sideways, opening the garment to the ankles in one action. I cast my eyes up and down her body and comment, "Hallelujah! Everything's here and in its proper place." My wife of fifty-three years wrinkles up her nose and sticks her tongue out at me as she hands me her nightgown. It, too, has snap fasteners up its entire front.

I should heed Self's warnings more, "Take it easy or you'll get yourself into trouble." He is correct.

I make an equally smart second comment, which I should have kept to myself as per Self's hint. "It's a shame to cover up all the nice scenery with a night gown!" This time she punched me in the ribs with her thumb with more strength than I thought she possessed. I let out a very loud, "Whoops!"

Almost instantly I feel a wet tongue make two passes on my ankle and then I receive an ankle bite. Latte, my wife's private bodyguard is doing her duty. She had been under the bed and has risen to the challenge. JJL often threatens me by saying, "I'll yell, and you know who will come running with her mouth open!" I don't know it then, but this reaction on Latte's part will become a part of her regular private security guard routine. It will be repeated several times in the future.

Chapter 7

Senior Sitting, Napping and Illness
I Can't Nap with Three Females

It's early Wednesday morning. It will be a day at home with no Realtor marketing meeting. I will be writing, painting as a watercolorist perhaps, working around the house and being a caregiver. The better JJL's health is, the more I can accomplish. Before I put my coffee into the microwave I feel a wet sanding of my right ankle. Latte is ready for breakfast. While two cats eat breakfast and my coffee is heating, I start to the bathroom for a quick stop. As I pass the bed, I check to find JJL's eyes still closed in sleep. Yes, they are closed, but her arm raises with one finger extended, her silent aspirin ordering procedure. Like Latte, she practices silent communication. "An acetaminophen?" I ask aloud, since her eyes are closed and, she would not see my confirming one finger.

"No, a migraine capsule!"

"Pretty bad?" My question gets another silent bit of conversation, a nod. This first report indicates it's not going to be a good morning. I remember a line on an old TV show, "When Mama don't feel good, nobody feels good!" In fact, not feeling good appears to be JJL's normal behavior, a MO typical of her last several days. Last night's sleep medication should put her back to sleep while the migraine medicine begins to function. I pour a little milk into my coffee before heading to the red platform rocker, knowing Mocha will soon join me for our quality time.

Leaning back and lifting my left foot to rest on the cat pedestal, I think, "It's nice to sit, even though I've been out of bed for only a few minutes. Is this what getting old is all about?"

"Try it and see if you like sitting," Self suggests.

I start to concentrate on why I'm enjoying sitting when Mocha arrives on the top of the upholstered pedistool with a flying leap. While a dog is supposed to turn around three times before lying down, she can find a satisfactory position with only one turn. This teen-age lover reaches with a foot to touch my toes, which are beside her. We silently communicate. This little routine is the same each morning. She glances out of the window beside her before lowering her head to go to sleep as I enjoy my coffee.

"She is your cat, just as Jacquie wanted," Self reminds me, "at least for these few minutes. When Jacquie awakens and goes to her recliner for the day, she will replace you as the favored person with both cats as you will be up and moving about."

"I was too busy during my freshman years as a senior citizen to take the time to learn to enjoy just sitting. I was saving that for an older age," I tell Self. "Now, heavily into the third trimester of my life, I find I enjoy sitting at this quiet time of the morning. I probably shouldn't make it a habit or I won't get much accomplished in the few years, or perhaps moments, I have left."

To myself, I vow I'll postpone advanced sitting until I'm really old. That's probably a silly attitude, but it will keep my mind focused ahead and my hopes alive. I have a lot to do each day. I need to make our estate easier for the kids to deal with when we're gone. I also need to continue with the housework and shopping, since JJL lacks the strength and the will to do them. I'm finding this work plus the marketing of the inspection business leave me little energy or time for my watercolors, even though I've cut out art association meetings and competitive shows. I am still taking the time to judge or jury a half-dozen art shows a year.

"You do enjoy judging, and you find it a great mental shift from being concerned about Jacquie day and night." Self seems to understand me rather well.

Self's right. I do need to be away from the constant necessity of monitoring Jacquie. In fact, our doctor has given me a medicine to take when I find my stress too high. I am practicing stress-relaxing exercises. Several professionals from the HMO have told me to back off and get more help, as fulltime care-taking becomes an affliction itself.

"Don, do you remember the number of hits you found when you typed the word stress into the Internet? There were several million and many were directed to caregivers."

It is not that Jacquie needs fulltime care, it is that one never knows when her problems will cycle and reappear.

We bought a care-giving insurance policy years ago. I have just applied to use it part time. Hallelujah! It reimburses us the cost of Jane's services. This lady comes to the house two half days a week to wash, clean and be with Jacquie when I need to be marketing.

"That policy was a smart decision years ago, " Self remarks. "It's a win-win situation. If you need it, it's worth the money you've spent on its premiums. If you escape the need for it, that is worth a lot however measured."

"Yes, and if either of us are required to go to a home that cost is also covered."

A newspaper recently stated that six persons of ten will need care, and only a few have it. Two thirds of Americans believe Medi-Care will care for them. It will, but only after their own resources are exhausted. Then the help is far below minimal needs.

I still have some coffee in my cup, and continue thinking about the piece I'm writing for my weekly senior writing class. "You find that association with others your age and the creativity involved are quite satisfying as well as relaxing, Don," Self notes. "Keep it up, it's good for you!"

In the quiet of the emerging day, my mind turns to the tasks ahead. Getting ready for the last trimester of life takes creativity as well as planning. For quite awhile I have been ready for a series of garage sales to shed some of our belongings. JJL has developed a desire, or rather has a need, to avoid people. It is hard to have a garage sale without people. I will haul a lot of things to a charitable group, or leave it for the kids to dispose of if I should go first. I'd hate for the kids to have to do that.

"In fact," Self reminds me, "Your Jacquie feels so ill most of the time that she doesn't want to think about the problem. You need to do as your Dad did. When your mother, who never threw anything away, wasn't looking, he would dispose of things he found in the basement. Now and then she would catch him, and the cold winds would return to their relationship. Remember?"

"Yup, I do."

The problem most people my age face is that they have never been old before. They aren't prepared for the challenges, or for all the nuances that affect living plans. Appetites, thinking patterns, desires, outlooks, needs and relationships can and do change. The challenge is that they occur differently in individuals. There is no software that guarantees a predictable routine. We have a neighbor whose wife is incapacitated. He walks her in a wheelchair for blocks. I silently bless him for the care he gives his invalid wife. The same problem has occurred to a couple across the street, and yet another lady nearby is developing Alzheimer's disease quite early in life.

"Care for the aging is a concern creeping into the homes in your aging neighborhood, Don."

Decades ago, most parents lived with children in their later years when they needed care. The grandchildren then learned about aging. Now many people have no such familiarity about problems of the elderly, and our faster life does not allow home care as a solution for many families.

"Don, your parents took care of Grandpa Andy for fifteen years before he passed away in his nineties. JJL's mother stayed with you for a number of years before going to finish life at another daughter's home. Now parents are often sent to rest homes. Some homes offer advantages, but too many have a number of disadvantages."

As I sit with my coffee before dawn, I'm wondering how to prepare for the end of a lifetime as if I can influence it. "I believe I can," I say aloud, causing Mocha to turn her head my way. That is important, and I need to continue to do it in a reasonable yet resolute manner. "I've done enough thinking for one morning," I tell the cat as I leave her and take my empty cup to the kitchen. And to Self I say, "There are other important things I like to do. Since JJL will sleep for two hours more, I'll do another of my enjoyable activities. I'll go for my walk and watch the sunrise." I grab my hat, open the door and say to the eastern sky, "To Safeway and the three-mile walk, here I come."

A hike is a delight at this time of day. I find many other people up and away from home, but instead of watching the sunrise, they are driving and must watch the taillights of the commuter just ahead in their first traffic jam of the day. I'll miss ninety-five percent of the miracles of the new century, but today I'll enjoy the miracle of its dawn:

birds greeting it with joy, fresh and invigorating air, and colors fresh off God's palette. "She's a great exterior designer! What a God!" I tell myself. As an artist myself, I can appreciate Her skill.

The next day I put in a number of hours before JJL wakens. No, she does not sleep later than the sleep prescription medicine allows. I awaken very early to spend several hours at the word processor. As I finish breakfast I have a little ache in the midsection, so I take a nap for an hour or so. When I stop dozing I find Jacquie walking past the bed. I beckon her to lie down with me. She settles a foot away from me, a comfortable distance so we will not bother each other. We are setting the stage for my purgatory-like experience ahead.

As we start talking, Mocha hears our voices and joins us, settling between our bodies. JJL starts petting her and the quiet purring lessens as the cat begins to nap. Then Latte hops onto the bed and surveys her mistress's lap. It looks as usual, so the feline settles crosswise on it and immediately tucks her head and legs into her typical sleeping posture. Now we have two people and two cats thinking about resting.

"I don't think this is going to work for long," Self whispers into my ear.

I have never been one to turn into a statue on demand. Something itches, aches or tires. I rotate my left foot, which is tiring of its position. Immediately JJL grasps my hand and pulls it hard against her hip. I peek out of the right half of my closed eye. She squeezes my hand and her best commanding eye is on me. Words are not necessary to translate the signal: "Be still or you'll awaken your cat!" Knowing cats can sleep a long time, and there are two of them, I say to myself, "Now look what you've done. You've tied yourself down for awhile. Self is right."

Almost daily, Jacquie reminds me, "Mocha is like her master. She cannot be still for a moment!" At that point as if to underline my thought, Mocha stands up, arches her back and turns around to put her back against my ribs, with her feet touching my arm. I dared to crack open my eye. Jacquie's head slants toward me. It is shaking, and an eyebrow is raised. No translation's necessary.

"Frankly," I whisper to Self, "I'm in the clear. The cat wasn't comfortable."

I wonder how Jacquie and others can sit or lie so long without moving. As a boy, I was always glad when it was time for a hymn at church or a funeral so I could stand up. The trouble was that they wanted to sing all six verses and I was tired of standing still by the fourth verse. Without any help from me, things become interesting and even funny. I am blamed.

I feel a tickle on my upper arm. I believe I know what is causing it and another tiny squint from my poorest eye confirms my guess. Mocha has a tickle in one of her ears. There are two-inch hairs coming from inside them and some of these hairs are bothering her. Unconsciously, she flicks the ear in her sleep and it tickles my arm. I find this funny and chuckle inwardly. Unfortunately, Jacquie's tight grip on my hand against an equally sensitive thigh picks up my silent inner vibrations. She can't squeeze harder, so she pushes her thumbnail deeper into my hand. An outward movement of her jaw, visible through my all-but-closed eye, slams me an ultimatum: "Stop it!"

I try. I'm always trying, and some say, "Don's very trying." Things go well for a few moments until I decide to take my mind off my little discomforts. I will do some of my stress exercises. I turn my toes upward in my shoes and point them towards my ears. When I can go no farther, I turn the toes under and begin pushing them as far from my knees as I can. Then it happens. My knee joint pops. Mocha isn't the only one who opens her eyes. Jacquie does too with both eyebrows raised. Her thumbnail is cutting deeper. All I can is say, "My knee." Whether she believes me or not, I close my eyes and try to think of another silent exercise. I try pressing my buttocks together, but decide that too, causes a movement to go through my body. I curtail all activity. That is painful, very!

Now we have a silent argument. I am quiet, having no idea how to relieve an itch, but Mocha must have one also and gets up to stretch. I know it isn't me causing her to stretch, but I get JJL's signal again. I can tell it without an eyelid this time. My head begins to itch, but as I begin to move my left hand up my side, I peek and find you-know-who looking at me. Since she doesn't approve of scalp scratching at any time, I change my mind.

Mocha never turns off her sonar, and her mind-reading facility has no OFF switch to my knowledge. I believe she picks up Jacquie's mental signals, and she stands to stretch one more time before going to Jacquie's lap for a facial by Latte, whom she has awakened. This is my opportunity to exit the situation, and I do so without delay. It is none too soon, as the cats get into a fight on Jacquie's lap and the feline beauty shop closes immediately.

"That could have been worse, Don. You got up just in time," Self smirks.

It is a good thing I am enjoying the morning with JJL as much as I am. We don't know it yet but we will go through a series of both short and long term medical visits before we find what was wrong with my Jacquie. It will be a long time before diagnosis and a means of dealing with the problem is found. In the meantime Self is giving rather good advice: "Do the best you can, Don. Your Jacquie's problem will find some resolution. Hang in there!"

He's right, but it will be many weeks and a lot of frustration. We are being tested.

Chapter 8

A Poor Start Indeed!
Things Change, I Love It!

The score in the first inning sometimes sets the stage for the final score. I hope that is not the case today. I hope the pattern can be turned and a rally will follow. The score so far this morning is one to four. I don't get the wake up call till nearly six, and I waken refreshed. That is my only score. My only Hallelujah!

A pair of aching shoulders scores against me in an hour to tie it at one-all! I fumble in the bathroom for a couple of aspirin when JJL calls for one of her strong painkillers. I can't find it. I check the medicine cabinet twice, then agree to help her out of bed. After retrieving her glasses I lead her to the cabinet. She is unsteady on her feet and the half-light of the awakening day hurts her eyes. She finds the prescription her first try. The drug name on the label "I" for the first letter, but I thought I had heard her pronounce something starting with an "E". If hearing and spelling had been on the application to enter this world, I would have failed and never been born! I am now behind one to three.

The fourth score against me is her announcement, "I still taste that awful rice from last night. I only ate a few bites of that Chinese chicken rice bowl." With declining health, she is not up to cooking from scratch most of the time. While I believe my cooking is great, I lose that argument on a regular basis. I realize I'm not Martha Stewart, but even Martha's cooking wouldn't receive a good review if JJL is not feeling well.

The problem is that her tastes have changed. She used to enjoy pearl onions. Now onions and a diabetic stomach cause her several problems. Having a super sensitive sense of smell and taste causes some people to become gourmet consultants. In my JJL, it has the opposite effect. Her dislike of the rice bowl, coupled with the misery and unhappiness of a migraine, predicts a bad day for everyone except the cats. I hope the prescription that starts with an "I" works well and quickly. Jacquie has had her quota of headaches this year.

"Don, you could celebrate if a migraine solution could be found," Self suggests. Solving the major headache problems suffered by so many people would certainly be a feather in the cap of any medical personnel making the breakthrough.

He is right and several months later I do. It's a medical blessing.

Now that her painkiller has been found, I can finish the trip I was starting, to the bathroom. The cats follow me. Latte makes a circuitous route behind the toilet, pausing beside a right leg for a pat or two before she comes to a stop on the scale to register her nine pounds. Mocha takes the direct route to rub against a bare left leg as she starts her conversation with me. Meanwhile, Latte jumps to the windowsill, to monitor any activities outside.

Later, I pull my cup of caffeine from the microwave as the aspirins begin functioning in my shoulders. Relaxing in the platform rocker I contemplate my day. Watching the dawn develop over a cup of coffee is always good therapy but there is no sun today. It is raining. "Can there be a dawn without the sun?" I ask Self.

"Check the red Webster book and find the if dawn means the rising of the sun."

It says, "The first appearance of daylight, not sunlight. It's the lightening of the sky. Such silly thoughts," I retort.

Jacquie's pain and her cranky remarks about the dinner I warmed last night, bother me. I remember that I, too, have changed and acquired afflictions that trouble and even upset her. To look at the other side of the ledger, I'm no longer the handsome prize she captured more than a half century ago. My trousers need a longer belt, and I am smooth where there once was considerable hair. I can no longer eat the rich food my mother cooked when I was a boy.

My inner partner brings back an old memory. "Remember how, after butchering a hog, and rendering the lard, your mother would fry apples with cracklings, the crisp bits of greasy fiber left after the lard had been boiled and rendered from them. This recipe, an attempt to salvage everything and waste nothing, is called scrapple. If cracklings were to have today's required food labels, the calorie and unsaturated fat levels would astound us. What a greasy staple."

I remember quite well. "Dad as a boy traded his good sandwiches with the Van Buren boys at country school. That poor family butchered a lot of hogs each winter, and they had lard sandwiches with homemade bread. Sausage was fried after the butchering, and links or patties were stored in crocks or glass jars with liquid lard poured into the container to keep air from the meat."

The great depression and dust bowl of the thirties created some strange recipes. We had a cucumber patch below a cattle tank that overflowed to water the plants. Mother used the cucumbers and onions she grew to make bread and butter pickles. I had butter pickle sandwiches for school that winter on homemade bread. We hauled a trailer of wheat to the miller to trade for sacks of flour. We ate a lot of homemade bread.

"Hey, guy," my sidekick smirks, "your most disappointing change of food relationship is with ice cream."

"Yeah, as a kid on the farm we had with plenty of milk and cream. There was winter ice on the stock tanks so homemade ice cream was a staple in our winter diet. In summer Dad would buy a block of ice when he went to town for sharpened plowshares, and we could have ice cream for a hot weather treat. I knew it would be Heaven on earth when I became old, lost my teeth and lived on ice cream. Instead, I became old, kept most of my teeth and developed an allergy to milk. Now, it's the Other Place on earth as I walk past the ice cream cases at Safeway. I used to know the locations of all the ice cream stores in the cities where I marketed our house inspection business. Now I no longer remember where they are or care."

"It's good you can eat a cone now and then but stay away from seconds for a week Don."

Memories are a great companion, but I must get busy. There's no future living in the past. While I have some age against me, I am captain of a keyboard rather than the skipper of a rocking chair. I still have time for rocking in the future. If not, so what?

It is time to help Jacquie to the bathroom. She uses a walker, but fell backwards out of it three times onto her head, so I grasp her arm as we travel. Oddly, she complains that the walker steers to the right even though the wheels are not steerable.

I need to start writing next month's Realtor newsletter, so I go to the computer, but not before Mocha races across the two desks to place her in position for petting. She, too, needs attention; in fact, she thrives on not only getting it, but also sharing it. She would be a good cat for a rest home, except she has not learned to stay away from walking feet, and could be a tripping hazard. There are projects in many communities where pets are taken to visit the elderly and shut-ins, with great rewards.

This lover, now an almost grown cat, walks over my arms and stops in front of the monitor with her fluffy tail in my face. "You are a nice cat," I tell her and oblige her with more petting. Then she lies down on her towel within my reach and starts her next nap. I do believe her aggressive demand for attention has been good for JJL, and may be responsible for my wife's sporadic better health and attitude. Attitude is a factor in health, good or not so good, I believe. I hope these short episodes of feeling better will continue. Little do we expect that things would get much worse in the not too distant future.

"What shall I put into the newsletter?" I ask, to see if Self can help. Realtors are salespeople, and while they know houses in general, they often appreciate suggestions about construction and maintenance that can be useful to them or their clients.

Since all of us enjoy laughing at other people's mistakes, I always include several mistakes we have found in someone's house under the heading, "OOPS!" Thinking aloud for Self's benefit, I begin, "I'll tell of an improperly placed toilet stool we once found. Most codes require twenty-four inches of open space in front of a toilet. This one had only six inches. To use it, one had to scoot the feet sideways, throw a leg over as if mounting a horse or sit sidesaddle. I'll also tell of a contractor who poured a patio over a septic tank, preventing access for later cleaning and servicing. The third OOPS will be the electrical switch plate glued on a wall to hide a hole in the wall."

The "WATCH FOR…" section is to help Realtors avoid problems in their transactions. One of my favorites is, "Be careful of remodeling or doing add-ons without city building permits." Improper work is often shoddy and even dangerous. Today's example is the homeowner who buried a long flexible tube in his back yard to carry gas to a brazier. The tube could develop a leak, or a spade could cut it, releasing gas. I'll also include a reminder to check that smoke detectors have batteries when moving into a new house. Children often borrow these batteries to power their toys, leaving no fire protection.

As some Realtors publish their own newsletter, I include items they may borrow. The Realtor can remind readers it is wise to not only insist a contractor obtain a building permit, but to withhold ten percent or more of the fee until the city has signed the final inspection papers. A lot of items in this section can be helpful to readers, as many new homeowners have been renters, and, like new parents, have little how-to or maintenance training.

I may restart a tradition I used several years ago, a motto or wise saying as the bottom line. When dancing with customers, let them lead! Is this one I like? Success is a marathon, not a sprint. I'll use it.

Looking out the window of my art studio-plus-office, I notice birds I feed are out of food. It is wet outside, but I guess that doesn't keep them from being hungry. I think there is an old folk saying, "If the birds are out in the rain, it will rain for quite a spell, otherwise they'll stay under shelter 'till it stops." I fill the feeders on the fence and put some millet and sunflower seeds on the ground. Finding it chilly I hurry inside to the newsletter. The top of Mt.Diablo is hidden in the clouds. Diablo is the Spanish translation for the Indian name for our resident old volcano, meaning Devil Mountain.

I go to check Jacquie. It's nearly ten AM. She is still asleep under the influence of her medicine. Latte has arisen from between JJL's knees and is paddling towards the dry cat food. I say "paddling," because she has a peculiar walk habit. I became aware of animal walking habits and foot placement in Professor Bell's Freshmen Livestock Judging class at college sixty years ago. He especially loved judging horses. He had coarse black hair and stood tall and erect. He would point with his stock judge's show cane to signal an aide to walk and then trot a horse away and back to the class. In his low, slow voice, he would critique each horse after we students had marked our scoring cards. A horse must move each foot forward in a straight line; otherwise its feet were said to be paddling. Hooves passing too close to each other could injure the other foot. It was a serious demerit.

Latte paddles with her front paws placed one directly in front of the other. If she were to walk through dust, she would leave three lines of footprints instead of two. If she were Professor Bell's cat, he would put a blue handicapped sign on her parking space, though she would lose her qualification for the sign if anyone were to see the way she chases Mocha under the piano, under tables and between chairs.. Just as Mocha has brought some rejuvenation to Jacquie, she has helped Latte loosen up as well. The older cat has become more active and more relaxed.

Mocha follows me as I return to my studio. I am standing near my easel to start a watercolor. Mocha hops onto the top of the computer case to watch me. A piece of paper left on the case does not provide solid footing. She slips backward and falls between the desks, tumbling through the myriad of wires and cables, with more noise than one would expect. It takes a moment for her to extract herself from the tangle of wires and cables and regain her composure. The mishap is not only unladylike, it is not in keeping with the surefootedness of the feline species. It will be one of her most embarrassing moments for quite some time.

I need to crawl under the desk to retrieve my "mouse" from the maze of wires, turn off the CD music and shut down the computer. There are also a number of papers and envelopes on the floor, which fell with her.

It's another day with a predawn wakening. After a few minutes, the microwave dings; "Your coffee is ready." I top the hot decaf with some non-lactose milk and carefully walk across the all-but-dark house to my early morning meditation center. I can't see in the dark like a cat, but living here thirty years has allowed my subconscious direction finder to become rather adept at guiding me unless someone has misplaced a chair. Barefooted several nights ago I step on a plastic Christmas tree ornament the cats stole from the tree last season to use as a toy. The ornament crunches and I jump. I am instantly awake. I'm not sure if that surprise is greater than stepping bare foot upon some cold wet cat food one of them recently dropped on the kitchen floor.

Sitting in the old red platform rocker with my decaf, I gaze out the window at the dawn nature is creating. Mocha arrives on her penthouse roof atop the scratching post and lies down ready for a session of petting and purring. We enjoy our quality time once more. I hope there is to be many of these, quality once mores. We both enjoy the habit. I find this relaxation with caffeine and Mocha's friendship finishes the wakening process and readies me for the day. In the summer of my life I was more objective oriented: lesson plans, budgets, retirement schemes and other schedules. Now I'm more tuned to subjectivity: touching, feeling, and petting (cats of course). I should have done this all my life. I recently heard a councilor for the aged say this is one of the larger needs for the aged, a need for being touched. Reading my mind, Self whispers, "That's true for most people regardless of age, Don. A handshake is all that's needed by some people while others like a hug. Watch the news and you'll see people in other parts of the world kissing a cheek of giving a quick hug."

It is still dark outside and damp, I notice, as I retrieve the newspaper from the front porch. The overcast is complete and rather low, suggesting some fog in places.

"It will be a day similar to your mood unless something changes, a nothing-to-brag-about situation," Self warns me. "Take your walk to Safeway for a fresh breakfast roll."

"Thanks. I'll work on my attitude as I walk." Breathing fresh air while walking can do wonders if the journey has a positive send-off. Later today I'll be distributing inspection reports and newsletters to Realtors in eastern Walnut Creek. I must plan an attitude metamorphoses if I am to be effective with Realtors today and also enjoy myself. Perhaps I should have made coffee with caffeine this morning instead of the unleaded kind!

Slipping into a jacket and stepping outside, I realize the wind is chillier than I guessed. I exchange my hat for a stocking cap and begin the walk again. It is becoming light as I walk several blocks of Colgate Avenue where I meet Marie, one of the teachers I had as a principal. "Hi, Don! How are you?" she asks.

"At my age, whenever you see me, you know I'm doing great!' I reply with a grin.

"You're a cheerleader type, aren't you? I am, too," Marie replies. "The world needs cheerleaders. Keep it up." She turns and goes into her house with the paper. I'm cheered by her remarks and my attitude begins to turn for the better.

"It was good to have a positive person like her in front of a class of sixth graders," I tell Self. Teaching is more than the three R's. We could add at least two more rs: Role-modeling and Responsibility.

Several blocks down the street I meet a lady with two miniature beagles on their leashes. They're pulling her in a running mode.

"How far do they have to go to give you all the exercise you need?" I ask her.

"Not too far," she replies. "On weekends, my husband takes his bike to walk them till they wear down. Coward!"

In spite of the damp morning, there are a number of people walking, including several sets of young ladies and a few senior couples. Probably a third of them are walking a dog. A number of people are in the habit of taking their dogs to the park where the dog can run free or chase a ball. Meeting upbeat people whose attitude is up and exchanging greetings with them is changing my mood. I have forgotten about the briskness of the air.

After paying for our almond roll and a head of lettuce, I leave Safeway and start the return journey. The sun appears through an opening in the clouds over the Altamont Pass. The crows that were flying west last night are now flying east, singly or in small groups. They, too, are going for breakfast. I note that the meadowlark's breast, so dull in the earlier drab morning, is now a brilliant yellow as the bird faces the sun. His trill as he greets the forming day is the final thing I need to boost my feelings. It's a great morning indeed! I'm ready to go marketing and be a positive force for our company. I enjoy walking into offices with a smile and receiving a return greeting, "Hello Mr. Larsen. How are you?"

A large yellow tow truck is sitting in a vacant parking lot I pass on the way to Safeway. I notice a similar truck in the store's parking lot. On the way home, I see a third truck beside the first one with the drivers visiting. Decades ago, tow trucks were parked behind a filling station or a car dealer's building for use when needed. Then someone would quit what they were doing and go to the accident scene. Now it appears to be a fulltime job, a sizable business. I often see tow trucks patrolling the freeway. These trucks are waiting a call, just like taxis wait and cruise in the big cities. Like vultures, these trucks don't cause problems; they exist to pick up the pieces.

I see a sheriff ground squirrel sitting atop his guard mound, watching for intruders. I wonder how long it will be before he is evicted from his domain. A posted sign states a large home improvement warehouse will soon be built on the site.

It is a little after seven as I walk near Jackson Avenue School. Parents are dropping their children to go into the pre-school-hour care. When I was the principal here, we had a rule of accepting no children before eight. Most dads were employed at the Lab down on East Avenue, and the mothers were homemakers. Now many parents both have work and to commute an hour or more to their jobs. The school is becoming even more of a substitute parent. We call this progress? Children waiting for school and parents sitting in traffic jams?

"It must be tough to play God with a winning hand, Don." Self is hiding under my jacket out of the cold. "Don't apply for the position of God! She can keep Her job, being the target of so much blame and responsibility."

Turning the last corner, I start downhill. My neighbor, Jay, is dressed in his biking suit and preparing to push off. "Have a good ride," I tell him

"I shall. By the way, Don, we will be going away for three days. Would you throw our newspapers over the side fence for me? I shan't want it to look like we're not home."

"Sure thing. That's what neighbors are for. See you later!"

It's time to go inside to shave and shower after reading the paper. JJL will be awake and we will have the roll I bought and our senior medicines. Then it's time to leave again, in the car this time: to deliver reports and newsletters again. I say to Self, "Remind me, I'm to stop by the pharmacy for those zero prescriptions Dr. Banda has now OKed."

As I pick up the pills, I give the youthful clerks behind the drug counter a puzzle. That is a must-do task. One young lady told me, "No puzzle, no pills!" I liked her teasing smile. Smiles are medications and they don't need a prescription.

I smile as I drive past the Lincoln Highway Garage, an auto museum dating to before the Lincoln highway became US 50 and ran past our farmhouse in Kansas. US 50 became Highway 580, which runs across the Western half of the nation. I remind my companion, "If those early engineers could see the road now as an eight-lane freeway with all the interchanges and fly-overs they would be wide eyed."

My merge with the westbound commute traffic is slow this morning. I'll stay in the slow lane. I find the majority of those entering the freeway move to the so-called fast lanes, which not only slows them, but also lessens the traffic in my right lane. In fact, I can often go for several miles at their pace. Driving in this melee means I need to keep my eyes only on the road and my neighboring drivers. I cannot enjoy the countryside I know to be green and starting to bloom in many areas. That can come later when I'm off the traffic jugular.

Stopping at a small realty office, I hand the secretary my latest word search puzzle. She asks me, "Mr. Larsen, how are you?"

"I feel like you look, great!"

I hear my Jacquie's voice in my head, "You should cut out that malarkey Don."

"I never lose an argument about how I feel," I reply to her silently. "They know me and smile. I like their smiles. Smiles make me feel good."

I then put copies of the newsletter into agent boxes and I'm again on my way to the next office. I'm greeted with a similar question and there is more smiling.

My answer may vary, "How am I? At my age, you know any time you see me you know I'm doing OK. I'm fine and you look to be in good health!"

They know it is a flippant remark, but you should see the smiles and relaxation that result. I am a pleasant break in their routines and we both enjoy a happy moment. I recently had a store clerk tells me, "From my side of the counter, we do not see enough smiles. Most people are too serious."

I am now farther out Ygnacio Valley Road in open countryside. There's little traffic and I can enjoy the countryside in bloom. The yellow mustard weed is bright against the green of the newest grass, and volunteer almond trees are also blooming. Some almonds have the traditional light pink blossoms; others are pinkish-red. A few appear to have double flowers. The dark trunks with light flowers silhouetted against the green grass are a delight to my eyes. The birds are also enjoying spring. They are on the ground, fences and trees, singing. The air is clear, and as I top a ridge I can see the beginning of the Delta and the hills across the great Sacramento River, with a backdrop of white wispy clouds. I should do a watercolor of the area.

A yellow light warns me to watch my driving. In an hour or so I will have finished my deliveries and greeted all the secretaries and a few agents. Then it is home. I have learned that several hours of marketing is enough or I will suffer from lethargy in the afternoon.

Self has noticed that result also, "Relax, Don. Enjoy the drive home. Then we'll see how JJL's morning is going." I had taken her to the bathroom, before I left and made sure she had water beside the bed. She would have gone back to sleep.

Hearing me come into the house JJL awakens. I help her up and to the bathroom. She wants to stay in a robe so I escort her to her half of the recliner and give her the morning paper. Then it's pills, breakfast and TV. The first signs suggest it doesn't look like a good day for her and perhaps for me either.

It is time to take the large tray of medicine containers to the table and start filling the week's daily allotments of medical necessities. Counting pills to fill a weekly container for an older person takes concentration and time. Doing it for two septuagenarians becomes an ordeal of nearly an hour, and a rest break is in order.

After a brief rest I start next month's newsletter. Thank goodness for spell checkers. If I needed to pass a spelling test before being born, I would have been aborted in early term. While I can remember words causing me trouble, I can't remember which of two ways is the correct spelling. The surgeon told me before the heart by-pass operation, "You'll feel better when I finish the operation, but your short term memory may suffer." He was right. It did. But my health is vastly better!

Jacquie needs an aspirin. I take it to her not knowing she will fall again and I'll be commuting to the hospital regularly in two months. Neither will I guess that two ambulances would be involved simultaneously to begin one commute in the middle of a night. Before long, our marriage will take on a different form and our lives will change forever.

I need to call my daughter-in-law, Donna, to see if there will be reports to deliver to Realtor offices tomorrow. One more female to give me directions: JJL, two female cats and a daughter-in-law. It's a good thing I love them or we all would have a problem! There are three reports for the next county.

Another female will be giving me directions about something not talked about in public.

Chapter 9

Rather Than Talk About it They Wrote Me
It's Your Turn the Letter Said

"Should I let them do this to me?" I ask Jacquie as I leave the house.

"Sure, no big deal."

I don't ask Self as he is smirking . He thinks it is funny.

It happens today but I got wind of it a month ago. I received a letter from our HMO with a first-class stamp on it. A first class stamp means I should open it. "We have been checking your records," this epistle stated, "and find that you are of the age to have a sigmoidoscopy and you have never had one. Please call 555-6277 and set up an appointment soon."

"What's a sigmoidoscopy?" I ask. We never had that word on a spelling list in grade school, and it wasn't one on a dictionary drill in a high school English class."

"Get your dictionary. You're a big boy," Jacquie said. A lot of help she is.

I look up the word in Webster and soon realized why the word is not in a school text. Little boys would have a field day giggling with that one. They would learn to spell it before they learned many shorter words.

The word deals with one's plumbing. As a house inspector, I examine the plumbing in a house, but only the outside of the pipes to make sure they aren't leaking or otherwise causing a problem. A sigmoidoscopy is an inspection of the inside of the body's biggest plumbing. The concept of a camera inside my body is not new to me. I had two angiograms prior to my heart bypass operation. At those sessions, a tiny camera on a wire was inserted into an artery in my groin and pushed through the artery up and into the heart. We were able to see the condition and clogging of the artery on a nice black and white computer-like monitor. The word sigmoid refers to the lower part of the colon, so I knew the inspection would not begin with the instruction, "Open wide and say ah!" It would be a far different procedure. Just thinking about it could give a person the shivers. Imagine being a sigmoidoscopist and having your children ask, "Daddy, what do you do at the hospital?"

"I work in the plumbing department." Bill Cosby could have a great response to this concept.

When I phoned the scheduling desk last month, I asked, "Can you schedule a sigmoidoscopy for me, please?"

"Yes. How about the thirteenth of next month? Is that OK?"

"Yes, if you tell me the thirteenth is not an unlucky day."

"Would you rather not come on the thirteenth?"

"No, schedule me. What time?"

"Four fifteen."

"Done. Do send instructions, though. If I am to go through the procedure, I don't want to botch it and have to try again. I want it correct the first try. Today I don't want to hear that old saying, If at first you don't succeed, try, try again!"

In a few days my instructions arrived. Jacquie read them aloud, "The day before the exam: Drink eight glasses of water and avoid any foods with seeds such as tomatoes, poppy seeds, kiwis etc.

"The day of the exam: Do not eat. Drink black coffee, tea or clear broth.

"Two hours before the appointment: Use two enemas and use at least two rinses with clear water or until the fluids run clear."

I wasn't pleased that Self also heard the instructions and was now helping: "Now you know what to do. We need to go shopping for enemas the night before."

We did and the drug store must sell quite a few, as the sales clerk didn't snicker when I brought them to the checkout counter. I remembered a boss my wife had who took an enema or two every time she had a cold, a headache or any other problem. The sale of packaged enemas must be rather commonplace. With the population growing, maybe we should invest in enemas rather than utilities.

Before starting coffee this morning, I recheck the directions. They say black coffee, so black it is. I attend the Realtor marketing meeting in Walnut Creek and arrive back in Livermore in time to make a pit stop before my writing class. I'm concerned that I will have inspection reports to deliver, which would interfere with my preparations for the HMO appointment, but a quick cellular call to Donna relieves my mind. She has lost the report inside the computer. To make matters worse, Jon had worked on it until three this morning.

As I come through the door from the garage after class, Jacquie has instructions for me. "Stay out of the kitchen. You are not to eat, remember?"

"I do remember," Am I reinforcing her personnel administration tendencies, or showing appreciation for her consideration of helpfulness to me? I decided to let the issue go unanswered. "I find it hard to sit beside you while you're eating," I tell her as I occupy my recliner.

"You can do it." Is she informing or ordering me to do it?

Soon, I start the sigmoidoscopy preparation. Going to the bedroom, I notice a large beach towel doubled and placed on the middle of my side of the bed. JJL is acting as my live-in nurse. I wonder if the procedure on me is causing her to forget herself and how badly she has felt the last few weeks. Before I get near the bed Mocha lands on it with a flying leap, runs to the towel and stretches out across it, claiming it as her own. As I kick off my shoes and drop my trousers, Jacquie brings the first syringe, already taken from its package and with its cover removed. She, too, has read the instructions. "Lie on your right side with your rump towards the edge of the bed and your knees drawn to your waist," she orders. She sounded just like a nurse yet she has had no training other than being a wife. Some things just come naturally to wives, I guess.

Bending over with the syringe she says, "Maybe you can do this easier than I can." She thrusts the syringe into my hand. I am right-handed but she has me lying on that hand. The free hand is my left one. This will be a challenge not only to do location scouting but also to squeeze the bottle until it is empty. To complicate the process, it is a backhand maneuver and I can't view the area as well as cats and dogs can.

"Patience, Don." Self is now also being helpful.

"Since this is an awkward procedure and I'm on my side of the bed, I'm glad you had the foresight of the towel," I tell Jacquie. I'm beginning to wish I'd purchased a number of units for backup in case I have a problem. I surprise myself and manage to have success with both halves of the task. It is now time to get up, move around and wait for results. I don't have long to wait. Enemas have a software operational program of their own, and leave no doubt as to the next procedure or process. The choices, as on a word processor, are delete or continue.

My resident nurse informs me I should lie down and use the second enema. Now that I am an experienced technician, the process goes more quickly. After the insertion of the first water flushing rinse, I show gratitude to my nurse, "Thanks for using warm water, Jacquie. I appreciate your thoughtfulness!" Two more rinses and the discharges are clear, so it is time to dress and leave.

The last time I was in the HMO pharmacy I picked up a flyer for heart patients suggesting a regular cholesterol test. Since it requires a twelve-hour fast, I have decided to stop to give blood for a cholesterol test while I'm at the HMO facility. The waiting line is short and the technician's needle is very sharp. My personal day of testing is going quite well so far, and I am nearly an hour early for the sigmoidoscopy. I have just seated myself after reporting to the clerk when a young lady sticks her head into the waiting room and calls, "Mr. Larsen!" The time for my exploratory expedition has arrived and I am casting off into a new experience. I will soon be a novice no longer.

I am led into a small room containing an examining table and a medium sized machine. There is a monitor on the opposite wall. The young lady introduces me to an operator at the machine, who tells me to strip from the waist down and then to lie on my left side on the table. I'm used to taking orders from women, so I grab my belt to do as I'm told. The lady at the machine dashes to the door. Before slamming it shut, she cries, "Wait to strip until I get out of here!" Is she modest? Does this septuagenarian male appear to be a threat to her, or is this clinic procedure? Self thinks this is funny and says, "All of the above."

An Old Man

I ask him, as if he knew, "What goes here? This is a rather intimate procedure, yet they act like modesty is to be preserved at all costs." I strip and crawl onto the table after finding a blue plastic modesty sheet to cover me.

There is a knock at the door. "Are you ready? Are you covered?" a voice calls.

I call back, "Welcome, come in!"

A handsome young fellow arrives, followed by the two young ladies. He gives me a big grin and a strong handshake. The girls go around behind me. I wonder about the significance of the big grin is as he approaches my backside. Am I too suspicious? Then my plastic sheet is flipped off me from toes to elbow, blowing away any modesty I managed to gather when I was alone in the room. To add insult to injury the video monitor is switched on, showing my backside in living color. Self can hardly contain his laughter. I found I have more hair on both sides of a very big magnified cleavage than I have on my head. Maybe I should consider some hair transplants. The problem is this hair is curlier than the hair on my scalp. "How would you explain that to anyone?" my none-too-silent inner partner asks.

"You may watch the screen if you choose," the camera driver comments as he violates me. I guess he didn't rape me, as I have given written consent to the procedure.

What follows is a travelogue without any sound. The instructions had stated there would be some air introduced to round out the colon to make the examination easier. As a result the colon is fully open, expanded and in full color. It reminds me of the lava tubes, leftover from volcanic eruptions, that a person can walk through. Moving through the tube is what the scope is doing. There are concentric rings with veining of colorful tiny blood vessels. It is a beautiful sight. It would make a grand geometric watercolor. My problem would be naming the painting. Perhaps Creation #1 would be best.

The scope goes up and down and from side to side as it rushes forward and is pulled backward. All four of us are looking for any strange formations, polyps, or nodules. We don't see any, thank goodness, and the guided tour ends.

"No need to take biopsies. Congratulations." The gentleman says this in a congratulatory manner. "You have the colon of a thirty-year-old."

The crew recovers my body with the blue plastic sheet. They leave me to use a tissue or two and to dress with an admonition of, "But wait till we're out of here." It is time for me to restore my modesty.

It is time for another, "Hallelujah!" The thirteenth is a lucky day for me. Jacquie is in better form also. Caring and worrying about me seemed to give her strength and stamina. I hope it will last.

Donald, You're In Trouble!
Jumpy Cats

Last night I was tired and went to sleep watching TV and reading. Today I have little pep, so I'll choose small type chores to do. I tell myself, it's OK to goof off as a senior, but only once in very long time. At this stage of life, every minute must count!

Jacquie has a different philosophy. "At this stage you should enjoy what life is left. Sit down and do nothing or read. Enjoy every minute." I don't think this is a sexual characteristic, as I see ladies who appear to go a mile a minute until the last. We didn't know it then that her days of rushing are ending.

I rest for awhile upon reaching home after flowing with commute traffic. I peeled a cheese stick, quite silently, I believe. However, Mocha who is asleep ten feet away raises her head, opens her eyes and sniffs the air before arising and coming to my lap to beg for a cheese tasting.

It's another day and my morning built-in alarm awakens me a little after five. I don't have much energy, so I go back to bed hoping for sleep. It is a futile decision but I enjoy the thoughts slipping through my consciousness. I appreciate a number of things.

I notice that the local recreation department is running an exercise class next door to our writing class for seniors. Outside that exercise room a health professional takes blood pressure and other tests once a month. A doctor is present. A doctor is present on several TV stations at the six o' clock and late newscasts not only with advice but also answering phone calls. It is indeed a great era to be a senior. My parents and grandparents saw the undertaker more often than an advisory health person.

At six I decide sleep has eluded me for another day and I arise. I take my coffee to the red chair and put a foot onto the cat tower just as Mocha arrives on it. While she is inspecting my sock, I remember a conversation last night about the practice of putting my foot here. "You are tipping and bending the tower," my spouse complains.

"The base is small, and it is sitting on a carpet that has some give to it. The tower is relatively strong," I reply. It is hard to win such argument, husbands have found, so the foot came off without continuing the argument. This morning in my solitude, I check my theory of its strength. The tower moves, but as a unit, not as parts. Hallelujah!

"Mocha doesn't mind the sway. She's a California cat, with earthquake sense in her software. She doesn't appear to notice the sway of the pedestal when it moves a bit," Self reminds me. I'll just have to watch that I don't put my foot upon it when JJL is present in the room.

Last night she had said, "Donald, get your foot off the pedestal before you break it." My mother christened me Donald and everyone in our small community knew that and respected her wishes. Don is not his name, neighbors were told. I was Donald in the small country school and church, but things changed when I went to stay with my maternal grandparents to go to high school. Mother had no influence at that school, and I became Don. Jacquie learned to call me Donald as courtship brought her into contact with mother. After marriage she called me Don again, until I ticked her off for some reason, and then I again became Donald, with all letters emphasized equally. Sometimes underlining was used as well. "Donald, get your feet off," is a message not to be ignored. The name, Donald, carries priority implications!

It was also **DONALD** in bold letters the other day when I was painting. She and the cats were in her recliner while I was busy in my studio with my watercolors. I needed to dry a damp passage, so I picked up and turned on the hair drier I use when painting. There was an immediate, **"DONALD, DONALD,"** from the living room. Since she used the priority title and repeated it, I believed there must be an accident. Had she fallen? I ran to her side. Her eyes screamed, **"DONALD, YOU'RE IN TROUBLE,"** with all words in capital letters. A head cocked to one side and lowered eyebrows carried back-up emphasis, with no chance of misunderstanding.

"You turned on your darned hair dryer and scared the cats." There are those darned personal pronouns in the second person. I am getting what would continue to be a message. It is to be a one-to-one epistle! "Mocha was asleep on my shoulder and went over my head, leaving scratches the whole distance! How bad is it?" She tilted back her head for examination. Before I could start my examination, she continued, "Latte was on my lap and she made a sprint along my legs on her way to the floor. Why don't you warn us when you are going to turn on your darned dryer?" That pronoun inserted in the recitation left little doubt as to whom she's addressing. It is a good thing I had clipped the cats' claws the week before, as few Band-Aids were needed. It would take time and visible repentance on my part to completely heal the wounds, both visible and invisible. I'll not use that dryer in the future, but I will have problems again with Jacquie in two or three weeks.

In the mean time I would become upset with another woman. Again it was communication. Some people listen with their mouths.

Chapter 10

Life Returns Today
I Have Communication Glitches

The October of one's life is when some of mankind's systems begin to fail or falter. There's one I'm glad hasn't failed me. I'm glad I still have the Old Man Alarm that sounds in the middle of the night. If the alarm were to fail I would have big problems. Now I get in the bathroom before I'm awake. What a reliable system! If the airline schedules were only as dependable.

By the time Nature is finished, my mind is completely awake and there is no chance to coax it back to sleep. "I've had a night's sleep," I inform Self. "It started early last night. Remember? I didn't feel good and used that as a reason to lie down. The British actors in the mystery we were watching did not pronounce their lines so I could understand them. That was an excellent reason to leave our double recliner."

JJL knew my feelings and suggested, no, ordered, "Go to bed." It seems that women gravitate from suggestions to orders as they age. If I were younger I would propose a research project along those lines. Women researchers would counter that aging men no longer respond to suggestions so orders are necessary.

Not realizing how tired I was, I relaxed on the bed and was soon asleep. In a few minutes my sergeant also gave up on the TV program. After she wakened me, we were soon under the coverings and I was asleep again.

This morning, after two aspirins to relax my arthritic shoulders and big cup of coffee to help me focus my thoughts for a writing class composition, I head for the red rocker. I look at the TV listings for four thirty and find it's all reruns from the black and white movie days or paid advertising. Forget it!

After a few minutes, I tell Self, "It's interesting that the warmth of the coffee and the attitudinal assistance of the chair help me mentally prepare to organize my outline." Before the coffee is finished, the shoulders are forgotten, and I go to the computer. I decide to call three pages of random notes onto the screen and cut and paste them into the bones of an outline I need.

"You've mused over those notes and now something appears to be coming together," Self responds.

I smile with inner pleasure that the composition is jelling. I'll push the composition to say that the busy senior who is accomplishing satisfactory things is a happy person. "Happy people live longer and, even more importantly, live better! I'll go to the library or the Internet to verify that statement."

The sun is almost high enough to flood the studio and shine into my eyes to obliterate the monitor screen. I turn off the desk light and get ready for my walk to Safeway. Pulling my miniature reminder pad from my shirt pocket, I see that I need to buy loose tea, white bread, a tube of breadstick dough, and cottage cheese. I'll be able to carry that load without trouble. Before I leave I start to pet Mocha, who is curled on her towel beside my keyboard, but she is asleep. It would be a shame to awaken her, but I'll bet her sonar will note my turning off the computer and leaving. It's time to go. The sun is in my eyes.

It is a nice walk. After turning east onto Colgate I adjust the brim of my old white hat to shade my eyes. The sun appears to be saying, "Good morning, Earth!" The earth responds, smelling fresh after a short nighttime shower. Cats are returning after their nocturnal hunting forays. A mourning dove greets the day with its low-pitched call. As a boy, I thought it was morning dove as I heard them in the morning. Then I learned mourning is the correct name; it refers to the cry's sorrowful sound. The night-singing mockingbird is finishing his repertoire, probably to the disgust of several late sleepers. He has his volume control turned to very loud, and his high voice is carrying from behind a house several yards away. The freeway a mile away adds its lower notes to the background of the morning symphony. The interesting thing is that there are no rest stops on the freeway's musical score. The low notes go on and on. I hear the sounds quite well in spite of not wearing my hearing aids.

I find these personal sound amplifiers to be a problem if there is any wind. The rushing noise they provide in even a light wind isn't desirable. I couldn't hear at class the other day so I turned the low background feature on and off with no success. The telephone switch change didn't help either. The tractor I rode as a kid didn't have a muffler. I think that noise may have started my ears' decline, although hearing people tell me, "Your hearing tests fit the norms of folks your age."

"Hallelujah!"

Self reminds me, "You have a problem understanding fast talkers."

"It's true." I often tell them, "You're talking faster than I can listen." The other day the young lady on the phone must have had a malfunctioning understanding chip, as she giggled after my comment and kept on rattling away telling me about the insurance she was selling. My comments did not register with her.

Another problem I have is dealing with people who don't listen. JJL and I were with a doctor last week where that became a problem. "My great toe was red next to the nail last night before Don cut the nail," JJL said. Feet can be a serious problem to a diabetic, which is the reason we were in the doctor's office.

It was obvious the lady wasn't listening, as she said, "The nail is cut close. Let it grow longer and see what happens."

"It was red for a day or two before he cut it last night."

"It's cut too short. Keep it longer! It's too short." She persisted along her line of thinking, in spite of my stopping her to repeat our concern.

Another day I punctured my thumb and put a bandage on it. Trying to count newsletters in a Realtor's office I commented, "My bandaged thumb bothers my counting these things. It's difficult to bandage a thumb."

The Realtor exclaimed, "You have it on wrong." She got a new bandage and pulled mine off. In a little while she continued, "It is problem to bandage a thumb and I can see it's hard to thumb through papers with a bandage."

I wanted to say, "You didn't listen to me."

"Listening is a skill to be learned," we told the people we hired for our inspection business. We also taught them: "Repeat what you think you're being told," to verify the communication link.

I found and pocketed a golf ball several days ago, and today I enjoy bouncing it as I walk and catching it with alternating hands. "Time and distance move faster with this ball," I tell my invisible partner, "but I must be a surprising sight to the motorists whipping by me."

"Some of them are interesting too," Self notes. "For example, there goes a van with a console between the front seats. The large dog found that to be a great place for the front half of his body. It allows him to have his head between his masters' heads and gives him a good view of the road ahead."

Before I get to Safeway I meet a fellow walking from a coffee shop with a large paper cup of coffee in one hand and a mitten on the other. I suggest with a big grin, "If you had ordered two cups you could keep both hands warm."

He smiles back. "I change hands," he says and we continue on our separate ways.

I note the seagulls are going seaward after last night's rain, hoping for a seafood lunch. I am surprised when Self announces, "Oh, there's a gull with only half of his landing gear retracted. His second leg is dangling. A one-legged seagull must have a very precarious life, as walking and swimming both are difficult and necessary for feeding. Poor guy."

As I walk by a newspaper in a driveway a large headline screams, "Try for Stadium Bonds." I've heard on the news that many cities are building new stadiums. It is interesting that these bonds pass, but sewer and school bonds go down in defeat. We often have a strange set of priorities. I'm reminded of Dad's story of a Quaker's saying: "All the world's queer but Thee and Me and sometimes I wonder about Thee!"

One of the houses on my route is being tented. That is a bad omen, meaning termites or beetles were discovered during a pest inspection. I don't see a posted guard, as required by law, but he may be in the rear yard. I'm reminded when Larry, our oldest son, was a pest operator. He went by a house he had ordered to be tented and saw no guard. It was twilight. He had been a referee for a soccer game and was still wearing his uniform. A neighbor saw Larry dressed all in black as he went into the back yard to find the guard. Thinking Larry was a burglar, the neighbor called the police. My son had to show his pest license to the policeman and the neighbor before the incident ended.

As I enter Safeway I walk by the serving counter where Chinese food is sold. While all counters, shelves and much of the floor space are covered with merchandise, this counter is empty. Self asks, "Don't Chinese eat breakfast? Do they just eat lunch and dinner? They could have oatmeal cakes or ham-and-egg rolls. What about scrambled egg soup or won ton waffles?"

Walking by the shelf of nuts I remember JJL's comment that I had eaten some cashews yesterday. It was true. I had. But why had JJL noticed it? Probably just practicing her wifely skills of detection and wanting me to know I couldn't get by with anything. That gives me an idea that may get me in trouble. I confide to Self, "I'll pull the same stunt on her that I pulled on her mother when she stayed with us years ago." A mother-in-law in one's house always creates actions to remember.

Hazel, my mother-in-law, had reached the age when it becomes necessary for a sex linked gene in some women to observe what happens around the premises. In fact, she had practiced and polished this skill by serving as a college housemother for several sororities and a fraternity. She did a good job of watching our street from our front windows. I suggested to JJL that we could rent elderly ladies to neighborhoods for crime surveillance and provide employment for seniors.

I had a box of candy on the counter and Hazel kept an eye on both the candy and me. The mischievous streak I inherited from both sides of my family broached itself, and I bought another similar box of candy. With the second box safely hidden, I began secretly replacing the candy I took to eat in front of her. The number of candy pieces in the box on the counter remained the same. A week later Hazel announced, "You are replacing candy but I can't find where you have the replenishments hidden!" I shrugged my shoulders, trying to keep a straight face and for once I won. It was hard to keep my face from giving me away. A second can of cashews are hidden from Jacquie. The plan is to put six or eight halves back when I take four. That should allow JJL to have some also and keep the nut level constant. The only problem is that JJL doesn't like being fooled, so I will have to allow the stunt to die an acceptable death rather early.

When I get home I go into the studio. Mocha is still asleep as I left her. Fifteen minutes after sitting down to the computer, I hear sound of the bedside TV. Walking into the bedroom I raise a hand with two fingers extended. Jacquie's eyes are barely open but her head nods. I bring the acetaminophen capsules and a glass of water with her morning medications. It is only eight-thirty so the heavy sedative pills wore off early, or did they? A few minutes later she is back asleep. When she wakens the second time, I will help her dress and feed her. Her health isn't improving.

A few minutes later I hear noises near the corner of the studio. Latte, is now standing in the litter box, attempting the covering detail by reaching outside the box to do the raking. She is a fastidious cat and does a lot of covering. After eating she will rake the rug around her feeding pan. I dropped a cookie crumb on the carpet yesterday and after deciding she didn't want it, she proceeded to rake the carpet in the vicinity.

The litter covering process completed, she goes to lie in the sun. She will follow the sun throughout the house. This afternoon she will be in the western part of the house. On cloudy days she locates the registers when she hears the furnace start to operate. She isn't asleep yet, she's watching the birds feed in the back yard.

Chapter 11

I Lost My Right Ear Last Night
Hospital Hi-jinks

A ten-year-old boy in the nearby city of Richmond had both ears chewed off last month when three pit bull dogs attacked him. When I awaken I discover I too have lost an ear in the night, my right ear, but I am fortunate. My "ear" is an electronic and plastic unit.

The boy's damage has kept him in critical condition for the past month. He'll live with a lot of help from doctors and concerned people around the nation. My ear problem should be easier to remedy. To regain my best hearing, all I have to do is await the arrival of daylight to search the house. Did I misplace my hearing aid, or did the Mocha bat it off the bedside table?

Mocha is recovering from the worst traumatic experiences of her short life. She is probably in the March segment of her life, and for the first time we had overnight visitors that stayed for several days. To make matters worse, two of the visitors were a pair of very loud and noisy boys known as our out-of-state grandsons, Lucas and Keiffer. Lucas is in kindergarten and Keiffer is a year younger. Both boys are very active, a real contrast from their grandparents Mocha grew up with. Mocha disappeared when Larry's family came in the door. The family stayed for several days and Mocha wasn't seen until they left to visit her parents in Berkeley. One night I once found Mocha by my studio counter, hiding behind an acrylic floor mat propped against the studio counter. The next day she had a different hideout and came out to welcome me as I returned to the house after dark when Larry's family had gone. She has not carried things about the house for several months, so finding and taking my earpiece must have been a trauma caused by the presence of the loud and active boys.

I take a breakfast break from the word processor, and then, now that dawn has arrived, I search for my ear. I can't find it. I look in the cats' water pan and in their litter box. I check the guest bedrooms, as the doors are open. No ear! Next break, I unmake my bed and search the bedding. Meanwhile, the cats race about and enjoy having the house back without strangers.

I think I'll call the HMO hospital and ask, "Can I buy a yearly or lifetime pass for my wife? You can tattoo a bar code on the back of her hand and just scan it to save filling out all the entrance paper forms."

"It could be done like a drive through a tollgate," Self suggests.

Yes, JJL is back in a hospital room after exactly a week at home. Tests, observations and routines register no conclusions so it's dismissal and home again. "Don, this is getting to be like a revolving door," Self whispers. Fortunately, she continues to pull her faux pas at the right time so medical can observe the happenings. That is in her favor. The latest incident coincided with our son's next visit three days later.

Larry, an EMT with Wichita ambulances, and his wife, Karen, a trauma room nurse, and their two sons return several days later to spend a few more days with us. JJL has been in bed all day but gets up to visit. An hour later we have some rather dramatic events.

"How have your days been since we saw you at my sister's ranch on the Fourth?" Larry asks his mother.

"Good and not too good," she answers. Larry and Karen are surprised that Jacquie's hospital follow-up appointment with Doctor Banda on the sixth found her weak and needing wheelchair transport. They look concerned when they learn that the nurse could not find enough fluid to take her blood pressure. "It took a liter of IV to allow the blood pressure instrument to function," Jacquie explains.

The hospital was worried about the possibility of dementia, so Dr. Banda sent your mother to see Dr. Watkins at Mental Health," I add, as Jacquie has not mentioned that.

"I was so disoriented that the examination was rescheduled for a week later. I also saw the diabetes nurse and the nutritionist," she relates. I am glad she remembers those visits. Her memory may be getting better, I think. I wonder if I will be proven wrong later.

"I took her to I-HOP for lunch, after she was finished at the HMO," I tell the kids. "She was weak, but properly oriented mentally. She had a lingenberry crepe before coming home to go to bed. Her problem seems to come and go. It's as if she drops a sheaf of loose papers and they fall in disorder."

As Larry moves to the chair beside her, I notice she is breathing differently: there is no rhythm. Catching Larry's eye, I point it out to him. He assumes a role he probably plays often as an EMT. After looking at his watch, he begins counting her breaths, which are becoming more noticeable. "Mom," he says, How does..." and he continues with several questions.

After awhile I interrupt the conversation. "Do you want to go to the bathroom, Jacquie?"

"Yes," she says, so I move her walker to her chair.

However, she doesn't reach for it. Ten minutes later Larry asks, "Mom, do you want to go to the bathroom?"

"I just did fifteen minutes ago."

'You're lucky your EMT son and his nurse wife are here," Self whispers. He sounds thankful.

Larry asks more questions, but JJL grows vague. She starts to answer each one, "No, I do not..." and then, with glazed eyes, stares across the room without saying more. After awhile, I decide it is time to check with the HMO. I call the advice nurse and hand the phone to Larry, figuring his knowledge of medical terms will be useful.

"Well my mother is..." He responds to the nurse's questions, and soon he is told to bring JJL to the ER or call 911 for transport. "Do you want the 911 route or take her yourself?" he asks me.

"Let's you and I take her," I reply. "Your observations as a medical person should be more helpful to them and get her more correct attention than my lay input."

"OK."

"Larry and I are taking you to the hospital," I tell JJL. "Do you want to go to the bathroom first?"

"Yes." We get her there OK, but she needs help to sit down. When she tries to stand again she can't. Larry moves behind her, reaches under her armpits and says as he starts to lift her, "Put your arms under her knees, Dad, lift them and back through the house to the garage. Lucas, open the garage door for Grandpa and me." By now she is burning with a fever.

After a quiet ride to Walnut Creek, I stop near midnight at the emergency entrance. Larry puts JJL in a wheelchair and hurries to the admitting room. By the time I have the car parked Larry has her processed through the first step and she is sitting in the waiting room. The second step is to answer a nurse's questions in a small room. "Who brought your to the hospital?" is one of the questions.

"Larry and Karen." This answer that causes the nurse to roll her eyes toward me. I shake my head, but the nurse is ahead of me; she understands I am not Karen.

"Take her to the waiting room, and her name will be called when the emergency room can take her." After fifteen minutes she is in ER room eleven, and getting settled in with blood pressure, temperature and blood sugar testing.

"Why's she here?" a youngish doctor asks as he probes her stomach for sore spots. "Does it hurt here? Here? Or here? If she's got a fever, then she has an infection somewhere. Probably a urinary infection. Those infections cause a lot of a woman's fever. Lean forward so I can listen to your lungs. She has pneumonia. We'll get some antibiotics in her through an IV and start fighting that, and re-hydrate her at the same time. She's quite dehydrated." Thinking he might want to have a little background on her other problems which might be linked to her condition, I start to relate them. The doctor informs me, "I'm here to react to her immediate problems and no others." Discussion ended. He leaves orders at the nerve center counter and disappears into another room.

"Don, he doesn't listen," my up-to-now silent Self complains.

"You're right. But if she's dehydrated let them take care of that. They'll watch her and find out more."

The nurse has trouble finding a vein. JJL's right arm has not recovered from the last war of the veins, and finding one is an almost futile task. Larry comments, "I have to insert needles while riding in the back of an ambulance."

"I'm glad I don't have to try that," the nurse says.

While waiting for the dripping IV fluid to re-hydrate JJL, am reminded that not all emergency visits are the result of illness. The staff is holding a chest X-ray toward the ceiling light and shaking their heads. The print is of a twelve-year old boy's chest. He had been eating popcorn at his grandmother's house while sitting under a wall shelf. A needle had fallen into his popcorn. He inhaled as he put some corn into his mouth causing the needle to enter his lungs.

Jacquie is responding to treatment and at five A.M. Larry and I come home, knowing she will be in the emergency room area perhaps for the rest of the day before a room in the hospital will be available for her. Mid-afternoon, Larry drops me back at the hospital while he and the family go to a living museum. When they return, I take the boys to a lawn area outside the hospital while Karen and Larry visit with and check on his mother. "She is much better, but she still made some remarks that were way off target," he tells me.

The next day is a bad day in several ways. A needle breaks and she bleeds over a good part of the bed before someone discovers it. She develops a bad headache that becomes worse after a vapor treatment. The vapor treatment is given a second time while I am there, with the same result. JJL is glad to see me and I am able to help when a nurse is not readily available. She still doesn't always say what she wants to say. She tells me, "The medicine they're giving me is making my urine softer!"

JJL isn't the only one with problems. Her roommate asks, "Where do I go? I gotta pee." I take the lady's arm to guide her to the bathroom, but JJL tells her there is a commode in her corner of the room.

I turn the lady around, and we are starting in that direction when a nurse arrives asking, "Where are you going?"

"I gotta pee."

"No you don't! You have a catheter. Get back into bed."

I wonder why I am writing this chronicle, and then I remember that just as JJL and I have never been in the October of our lives before, neither have our kids. Larry and his Karen are in the medical field, so they have considerable knowledge of what happens with the elderly. Jon and our daughter Karen, not being around the elderly much, might benefit by reading the experiences I'm recounting. September and perhaps the October of life can be a great time for many people, with cruises, trips, golf and other interests. Late October and perhaps November present different health challenges, we're finding.

I tried to make yesterday an interesting day for Rosie, the elderly lady in her November, to whom I've given the tennis balls and turnips in the past. I plant them in her lawn or hang them from the lemon tree just outside her kitchen window. I took a great grandson and two grandsons to deliver some more turnips to her. I directed them up the street to her door where they were to ring the doorbell and present their gifts. We generously give little surprises in the spring months of a person's life, but such attention can also help an elderly individual in many ways. In today's society, many of the elderly do not have family nearby to visit with them or befriend them.

My sharing of turnips is not all to the good, as I find out this morning. I see a middle-aged neighbor walk by so I ask her, "How did you like the turnips I left on your lawn?" She had told me a week earlier she liked turnips when I asked her if she wanted some.

"Did you leave those on our lawn? I saw them and thought our crazy new neighbors put them there. I was scared, so I cut them up very carefully. I thought they might be bombs. I'd better call Bob at work so he can stop worrying too."

I find this fascinating as Bob works at the huge research lab known to protesters as one of our nations bomb factories.

"You win some and you lose some," Self whispers.

Tonight is a celebration for a neighbor girl going away to college. She will receive a lot of attention. The elderly need noticing also. It's not the turnips or tennis balls I slip the old lady that make her day. It is the fact that someone stops by to notice and listen to her that breaks the monotony that is ever with her. Yesterday I saw her folded newspaper on her driveway, so I stood it on one end and walked on. She'll grin to herself knowing I paid her some attention. JJL's sister Maurine tells me some fellow in her town in Kansas picks her paper from the lawn and tosses it onto her porch as he walks past. Sharing and good deeds are perhaps universal, or should be.

I shave and dress before checking to find what kind of a night JJL had. I take her my first kohlrabi and a little lemon tomato. Perhaps it is the first time for that type of bouquet. I'll pick one or two of her favorite lilies tomorrow.

Oh yes, I find my ear. Mocha had pushed it between the legs of a bedside lamp. Our quality time is special this morning. She places herself on the bed beside me before I arise. She then comes to her pedestal for petting as I go to the rocker with my coffee. She soon hops down into the chair beside me and is so happy she has to rub against my hand. I all but spill my coffee. What a lover!

"There's no question whose cat she is," Self `confides to me.

When God created the world, I think She gave mankind pets as a segment of the healing arts. I do believe JJL has improved since we adopted Latte and Mocha. We both laugh a lot more than we did before. She gives the cats a priority over me if there is any question of their welfare in her mind. For example, she says, "Don, change Latte's water. She likes to have fresh water." I think having her small water pan refilled when empty is sufficient. I've a notion to tell her Mocha likes her water brewed for a day, but decide not to even think it loudly. By then I have received corrected instructions, "Not tap water. Use the filtered water we use!"

Jacquie tells me she is not the only older lady with problems. Her hospital roommate is an alcoholic and has learned quite well how to stash and hide her treats. When this roommate walked into the hospital after a long ambulance ride, she had a number of cookies concealed under her robe. While she was settling into the room, a nurse came in, her eyes following a small line of colored spots on the floor. It seemed the new patient had a container of ice cream under her robe as well as cookies. Shades of Hansel and Gretel. The ice cream was melting and it dripped to the floor, leaving a sticky trail of evidence. Besides asking for something sweet every time a nurse entered the room, this patient goes on raids to the unlocked snack stock room across the hall. On one such raid, she walked past JJL's bed with her gown open exposing most of her backside. With a jerk of her head over her shoulder her eyes met mine and she told me, "Sorry about the view, but there's nothing but butt back there."

My pushiness is to pay off, I find. For four days, I have been asking any health professional I see, "Why can't my wife swallow most food?"

The floor doctor finally says, "The ear, eye and throat doctor is on the floor and will be by to look at her throat."

"Hallelujah," Self shouts in my ear.

This medic soon appears, but he doesn't look at her throat. "I hear your sister and mother had a swallowing problem late in life, so I've scheduled an evaluation for you tomorrow morning. If needed, I'll dilate any constricted part of your throat," he says, and leaves.

Now I think we'll find out what a technician meant yesterday when the upper GI exam was stopped and the examining device withdrawn. I wasn't there but the examiner stated, "No use going any farther, I've found the problem." The episode was over with no explanation, or, perhaps JJL felt too ill to ask or to remember if she did ask.

Self's mind is working like mine. "She was probably told but doesn't remember. Don, you had better keep your ears open to find out what it is they found."

"Great," I tell my wife. "It paid me to be pushy this time. We're going to get some action." She sticks out her tongue at me and wrinkles her nose. She seldom gets that way with anyone but me. It is time for another IV.

The nurse can't find a vein to insert the needle. "I'll get the head of the ER room to do it. ER nurses are the best in the hospital," she says. That lady arrives, and after examining both of Jacquie's arms, elects to call the head of the department to do the insertion.

He is soon there, and after a careful search, he finds a vein successfully. "Whew," he says.

My wife's next treatment is one she will not forget even with her memory problems. She still says, "Never again! I'll die first." An ear, eye and throat person puts a tube in her throat to stretch the narrow place the technician had found earlier. "They had to hold me down!" she tells me when I arrive to visit. "I've never had anything hurt as much. It was awful."

The throat wasn't the problem, we are informed later. "It was the constriction at the bottom of the stomach that needed massaging," the specialist explains. "If that massaging isn't enough to give you relief, come back and I'll do some more," he promises.

"You'll never see me again, regardless of any problems," she answers. "And that wasn't massaging, regardless of what you call it." Her eyes underlined her message. He got her meaning.

Self snickers, "It's been years since I've heard her tell someone something so strongly! She's serious and he knows it."

Later in the day, she is released again from the hospital. As we leave the room, Jacquie and I see her roommate searching Jacquie's lunch tray for any uneaten sweets.

We say goodbye to the personnel at the nursing station, and even though it is summer, I added with genuine feeling, "And if we don't see you again, Merry Christmas and a Happy New Year!" I wanted to be optimistic. I will be proven wrong once again.

In the car, Jacquie says, "Home, James." We both hope she wouldn't have to return although we do not know what causes her problems. The next step is to set up a post-hospitalization follow-up with Dr. Banda.

Our ride home is like a nice Sunday afternoon drive. We are traveling against the traffic flow of weekend vacationers. There is a high count of boat trailers headed west and back to the Bay Area. JJL begins to worry if the cats have missed her. "I'll bet Latte will lick and nip me. Then she'll go off to ignore me as punishment for leaving her." Sure enough, that's the way her homecoming occurs. We find several photographs have been are knocked over, further evidence that the cats had been unhappy and lonesome.

Mocha is in a more congenial mood than Latte. Or is she just hungry or curious? Jacquie asks for a stick of cheese and opens its wrapper without apparent noise. Mocha's nose-and-ear radar picks up the operation and she is immediately upon JJL's lap hoping for a tidbit, which is soon given to her. Looking at this drama, I say to myself, "I hope our routine settles down to normal-whatever that is. I have been wrong other times when we came home from the hospital. Will this be the end of it, even though we have no definite diagnosis?"

It is then that Jacquie, coming from the bathroom with her walker, asks, "Hadn't we better get ready for my appointment?" She has no appointment today. Her eyelid cancer surgery is several days away. We hope that it will be a routine procedure, just as a little nose cancer removal was several months earlier. The day we learned the nose lesion operation had been successful, we learned our daughter was to have a cancerous breast removed and her husband was to have a golf sized tumor removed from a kidney. The operations will occur in the near future.

"If it's not one thing it's another or in your case, Don, it's several," Self sighs.

"So we'll cross our fingers," I reply. We had no idea of the cancers around the corner nor are we sure of JJL's problem yet.

Chapter 12

A Lull Between ER Visits
I Am my Own Assessor

We should be alarmed. Why can't, or don't, we take time to monitor ourselves, as we should in our journey through life? Oh yes, we do check our watch to see how much time we have before our next demand, and we look at our bank balance printed at the bottom of the ATM slip. It is easy to blame the fruits of civilization for encroaching on our time for reflection and thinking. Before portable radios it was easier to reflect when fishing or just sitting on the front porch. The horse of yesteryear could walk the buggy home, we didn't have to listen to traffic reports, and we could think. Having those times to ourselves is still possible, but we must program them.

I enjoy sitting in the dawn with a cup of coffee or tea, reflecting on what is happening in my life and considering what I can do with what is left of my shortening future. A walk as dawn breaks is one of the greatest delights of my elder years. The fresh air and the beauty of the awakening day set a stage for my now alert mind and memory. I am meeting more people, both young and old, like me, people who enjoy the opportunity to renew their minds and bodies by walking at this time of day. I notice smiles on most of their faces. The other day I caused a smile for a middle-aged lady, and myself as well, as we stopped to talk. She looked me in the eye and said, "Your fly is open."

I reply, "You sound like a wife!"

"I am." And that is when her smile occurred.

Squirrelly, an older neighbor whose eyesight is all but gone, says, as he pulls flowers along with weeds from his daughter's flowerbed,

"Don't ever be ninety-five, it's awful." Hearing that, I vow to enjoy each day before ninety-five and not wait for later promises.

"Don, enjoy your beautiful October of life and think about how you can maximize the rewards in your days of November should your calendar last that long," Self advises me. "Take a lesson from Dr. Devnich. She collects stamps, writes on her computer and attends classes at ninety-six." November slipped up on my JJL like a midwestern storm, quickly and without much warning. It crowded out most of her October.

I suspected Jacquie was approaching her November of life when she asked me on an overcast day in July to turn off the air conditioner and turn on the furnace. I remember my grandparents having body thermostats that differed from mine. Other signs now begin to fall into place to warn me of her changing life. Her interests are lagging. She will no longer go to a store other than a grocery store, and that, only occasionally. I am buying her clothes. At first I thought it was simply "Aging Wife Syndrome," but it is as if she realizes some of her systems are slipping. She shows her alertness in other ways. It is interesting to note that, while she cannot focus sufficiently to read a book after her eye surgery, she can spot a single strand of spider web on the other side of the room.

Our bodies are not like that delightful poem of Oliver Wendell Holmes, "The Deacon's One-Hoss Shay." This buggy is built so each part is of strength equal to all others. No piece will wear out before any other segment. "It will last a hundred years and a day," the blacksmith promises. The third owner, a deacon, is on his way to church when the hundred years and a day arrive. Everything breaks at once and the deacon finds himself sitting on the road amidst the pieces.

As we age, many of us begin reverting to our past. Perhaps my wife is reverting to her prior need to be alert as a mother of children. This may explain why she's becoming more aware of what I'm doing and has a need to instruct and supervise me. Self sticks his nose into my thoughts: "Yeah, Don, but maybe now you need more supervision than you did."

It started with simple things: "Don't chew that aspirin!" Or, "Where are you going now?" I explain, " I want some water." She gives me permission with an "OK." The next time I arise from my chair, "Now where are you going?"

" I drank too much and now I need to go to the bathroom." She again blesses me with an, "OK."

Squeezing my hand while we're out walking in the evening, she instructs, "Don't say anything," when a neighbor across the street comes out of his house to his car. As usual, she doesn't want to talk to anyone. "Are you awake?" merits my affirmative reply, but she informs me she heard me snore. She needed hearing assistance, and bought hearing aids several years ago. She is not wearing them now. Perhaps her need to hear me snore or chew an aspirin has exercised her hearing enough that it's become more acute!

She's a TVwatcher of the professional class. One evening when she's watching her choice seven o'clock program, she informs me, "You're not giving the story your full attention." I thought I could let my thoughts run to a writing class project that I need to polish. She's noticed that my head is pointed at the red chair, rather than the TV set. If she were watching the program, as she should be doing, she wouldn't notice my upturned eyes. She is playing Jessica Fletcher again, I decide.

Perhaps the need to be in control is not an aging feminine characteristic. It may be an aging attribute common to both sexes, but I have lived with very few older men so I can't verify that guess. My paternal grandfather lived with us when I was a boy, and his eagle-like eye was on everybody and he disapproved of most of what he saw. However, when I stayed with my maternal grandparents while in high school, it was my grandfather who was watched and corrected. "Henry, reach your coffee cup this way and I'll pour you some fresh! Stop shaking the cup, Henry!"

"I'm just trying to keep up with your feebleness, Mom," he'd say. He was hen-pecked. Grandma was the CEO not only in the kitchen, but also throughout the house. Perhaps it is just a case of one partner reaching seniorhood before the other and settling into the coaching or administrative role.

A change of leadership roles will explain why putting together our jigsaw puzzles has changed from a joint effort to one when JJL issues rules on how puzzles should be worked. Certain areas are to take priority while others must wait. I try to be in the middle of a good book when I set up the puzzle table for her.

"Don, you now know why it is older men who become ambassadors to foreign countries? They have learned how to keep their mouth shut and when to speak." I should stand Self in the corner for such remarks.

I know JJL loves me in spite of her tendency to award me points and penalize me as if I were in a sports competition. Which brings up the question, "Do some aging couples grow apart as they begin to need and depend on each other more?" I believe it is possible. I don't think we are growing apart because I notice that each of us, in the course of an evening of TV watching in our double recliner, reaches to grasp the other's hand. It appears that we are both narrowing our sphere of interest but including the other more.

In the past, I would ask her to ride along on a nice day as I marketed our company newsletter to real estate offices. "No," she'd reply, "if you're going to deliver a report, I'll go, but not if you're going to market with your newsletters. If you are delivering newsletters you go to more offices in a town and I have to sit longer." Now that she is ill and can't be left alone, she volunteers to go with me. She realizes her problem and her dependence on me for help, a great tribute I appreciate and a great step for her.

"Will you go with me if I go marketing?" I ask one morning.

"I thought you would never ask me!" she replies. Am I surprised! I think her going with me is like my choosing to not work jigsaw puzzles with her, a matter of respecting change.

In early June when tests indicated Jacquie's nose cancer was all removed, young Doctor Cee said, "I recommend Doctor Right for the surgery to remove the little cancer from your lower eye lid.. He's in our Contra Costa facility."

"Why don't you do it here?" I ask. "You got all the tissue from her nose."

"He has a better hand with a scalpel than I do," she replied with a knowing smile. I like this kind of honesty.

We met the doctor for consultation but had a problem with his question when the operation was discussed. "Do you want me to take what I think is the whole tumor and then stitch the incision shut? That way you can go home after an hour or so. Or would you prefer to wait while the tissue removed is checked to see if I have to go back to remove more?"

Jacquie looked at me and her silent voice asked, "Don, what shall we do?"

Why do we have to make your decision? I thought, but aloud I said, "Doctor, why do you ask us? You're the expert, not us!"

"When a patient is over eighty, we just remove the tumor and send the patient home, as this type of cancer grows slowly and generally will not be a problem to the patient ever again," he replies. "When the patient is under seventy there is a good chance it will grow back and have to be removed again. Mrs. Larsen is in the seventy-to-eighty-year range, and it is a toss-up from a medical standpoint."

Turning to my wife, I responded for both of us, "Since she's going for another thirty or forty years, take the longer procedure, Doctor."

"We'll still be finished by noon, even if I have to go back to remove more tissue," he assured us.

Today is the day and her appointment at the hospital is at eight A.M. Her medicines usually keep her asleep until nine or ten, so getting up at six is a challenge for her. We leave early due to the commute-crowded freeways.

Our timing is off, and we arrive quite early. As we sit outside the appropriate door, a friendly man emerges and comes to us. We visit and find he is part of the team that is going to remove the malignant tumor from Jacquie's lower eyelid. "I'm the person who will stain the removed tumor, freeze it and examine the slices microscopically to see if all the tumor has been removed," he tells us. I have trouble with that concept. It seems to me that one would look at the place it came from to check that it was all gone, rather than looking at the removed part.

The eye has been bothering Jacquie, so she is looking forward to the cancer's removal.

With the paperwork quickly finished, we are taken to the tiny operating room, which is equipped with only a table for the patient, a small machine and a chair for me. Once Jacquie is on the table, an electrode clamp from the machine is attached to her leg. After the red-headed nurse swabs JJL's eye socket with a deep yellow disinfectant, the doctor proceeds with a local anesthetic to the eyelid. In a moment, he takes a fountain-pen-sized electrode also attached to his machine and begins to excise the cancerous lump.

"You goin'ta watch this Don? I think I'll close my eyes whether you mind or not," Self mumbles.

"Go ahead." The last thing I want is an upset inner Self.

While I am watching the surgery, Jacquie announces, "I smell smoke."

"That's right, you do," the doctor answers. The tiny blue, three-eight's inch arc from the machine cauterizes the flesh as I remove the growth."

"And I can see a tiny wisp of smoke rising," I add without thinking it might disturb her, but it didn't. I notice the Doctor's nurse setting up a lady in a similar room across the hall, so I observe, "There must be quite a few operations of this type."

"Yes, they are quite common," he answers. The fellow we met earlier comes into the room. As the doctor's tweezers lift the removed tissue, the technician holds out a tiny vial to receive it. As the technician leaves for his lab, the doctor covers JJL's eye socket with a fold of gauze. Preparing to go to the patient across the hall, he says, "I'll be back in about an hour." Our waiting consists of her lying on the table while I held her hand and described what had happened. She had no pain. As he returns he is met by the assistant we met earlier and they have a short discussion. Doctor enters the room and as he removes the gauze, informs us, "I need to remove more tissue." As he sits on his small stool he bends over and picks up the little electronic surgical tool. Self again closes his eyes. After the next testing, we are assured, "All the tumor has been retrieved."

He next measured the length of the missing lower eyelid tissue before he inks an ellipse onto her upper eyelid to mark the skin that is to be used for the skin graft. The little tool slices the skin from this upper eyelid. This tissue is transferred to the lower lid and sewn in place, closing the gap left when the tumor was removed. The upper gap is drawn together and sutured. Both wounds are given a liberal application of ointment. After taping a metal shield over JJL's eye socket, the doctor instructs me, "Replenish the salve four or five times a day, and I'll see her in two weeks at my office." He bids us, good bye and goes across the hall to work with the lady on that table.

"Self, you can uncover your eyes now."

Both of the wounds heal to the point of being invisible and the doctor is pleased. We are very satisfied but what about the other cancers in our family?

Chapter 13

What About the Other Cancers?
Karen, Our Dynamo

Tuesday's schedules have been the same for a number of years: I arise early and am on the freeway by seven for the eight o'clock Realtor sales meeting in Walnut Creek. Merging with traffic is not difficult this morning and I stay in the right lane on the two freeways I use. After listening to the first of the traffic reports, I change to a light classic music radio station to relax and to enjoy the ride. Years before so much traffic, I used to enjoy the scenery. Now I must watch the road and other vehicles but I do notice a large housing development starting on in a roadside pasture.

This reminds me of our daughter Karen, who is deeply committed and involved in the issue of preserving agricultural land. She has been hired to head one organization for this purpose and also manages a related group. She and her husband live on a cattle ranch amongst the windmill generators in the Altamont Pass east of town. She was elected president of the California Cattle-woman's organization and her husband, Darrel, served as the vice-president of the men's organization before becoming the current president. This meant they travel a lot to state and national meetings and conventions. As a result we have seen little of them lately.

To most women, this would be a problem if fighting cancer. But instead of fitting her schedule around a mastectomy along with radiation treatments, she fitted the medical work into her schedule and proceeded full speed ahead. Because her mother was not well, Karen kept her and Darrel's problems to herself. Darrel had his lump removed without major surgery and her operation went well without our involvement.

She did stop by several times to show her new wig, her head without hair and give us up-dates and even a laugh or two about the hairless condition. Karen and Darrel drove to Stockton early one morning to fly their plane to southern California for a conference and meet the governor. As they approached the plane she remembered she didn't have her wig. There was no time to return to the ranch for it. Darrel flew south and she met the governor bareheaded. She had her own hair when on the front row of the National Cattlemen's convention and President Bush looked down at them several times. Their responsibilities have taken them to Washington for a week's lobbying two different years. When invited to spend an evening at a California senator's new home one evening, Karen was at ease, far different than her mother who is not comfortable with strangers.

Distance has passed easily as I think of our daughter. I turn onto the second freeway. Self who has been enjoying a lively piano composition on the car radio but also following my thoughts, comments, "It was fortunate she and Darrel met that doctor from Stanford at a cattle convention. Somehow he found out they each had cancer and he opened doors to the university's resources."

"They were well prepared for the operations when they occurred. The procedures went well and we were told of them afterwards." I had reached the Rudgear exit to town and my mind turned to traffic requirements.

Putting on my Larsen House Inspection nametag I took my word search puzzles into the hall and positioned myself to greet Realtors with a smile and a puzzle. I enjoy this routine. I find I feel more alive after smiling and greeting people for the half-hour before I leave. Reading my thoughts, Self adds, "The fact that several who don't know JJL, ask how your wife's doing is also a boost to you."

"Yes. I've noticed these short times seem to meet a social need now that I've had to curtail some art activities and Karen and Jon are almost too busy to spend much time with us. Self, when I was a kid before television and e-mail, families used to do more visiting." The meeting has started and the Realtors are using a promotional vocabulary to describe the houses for sale. As inspectors, we use a different vocabulary to describe the same houses. I grab a foam cup with coffee to enjoy as I start home.

A KCBS traffic report is favorable for my trip back to Livermore and I merge amongst southward bound travelers. As I switch to music, Self asks, "Do you remember when Karen was born? It was in different weather than this."

"It was January in Kansas with subsequent blizzards. Karen, like her mother and siblings, was a ten month baby."

"Yeah! You took JJL to town to stay with her folks rather than risk ten miles of country roads in a snowstorm."

"But that wasn't the end of Karen and the winter conditions. We had to take her back to town to see Doctor McGee about her infected navel. I slipped off the icy road into the ditch. I had to walk to Remple's farm to borrow a team of horses to pull our Ford V-8 back onto the road. We soon had other problems develop with that road."

"Like that time you and your dad took a tractor and trailer to town for a refrigerator and had to come back through the fields because the roads were too bad even for the tractor. Why did you need a refrigerator in January? That house was cool enough to keep things from spoiling."

"You're right, it was cold. After our evening meal in the kitchen we let that wood stove die down while we went to the bedroom where we had our oil heater. The water bucket and the bucket catching sink water had to be emptied before we went to bed or they would be frozen in the morning. We bought the refrigerator to keep Karen's formula from freezing." I also reminded him of our putting bundled Karen between us as we crawled in bed fully dressed one night. Our oil heater was turned up as high as we dared.

"And then you ran out of fuel oil the next day," Self reminded me.

"I called the fuel dealer for oil delivery. He was about to turn around eight miles south of town as the road to us was impassable for his truck, a road grader appeared. Hearing of our plight the maintainer operator produced a chain and towed the fuel truck the two miles to our farm. We were saved and Karen was kept warm."

"But it was not always cold on the farm. Remember the spring after Karen led her little brother, Larry, around with her to kill box elder bugs?"

"She would point to a bug and say, "Ugh," and he would raise a small foot to step on the insect.

I'm so carried away with memories that I all but miss my turnoff into town. I had started to remember her piano and academic successes. She enjoyed attending college and went on to marry the son of my principal.

Back in Livermore, I call Donna to see if she has any inspection reports for me to deliver. She does, "One to Danville and two to Walnut Creek. They're ready now, Dad." In a few minutes I'm repeating my miles west and north.

As I merge between two large tractor–trailer trucks I soon find Self hasn't forgotten Karen. "Boy, what a life she led for several years after they got out of college."

He's right. Darrel was recruited to manage a large ranch on the shoulder of Mt. Hamilton. This spread was a tax shelter by a Silicon Valley executive. Darrel was hired to turn the ranch into a profitable spread. The terrain was so rough our son-in-law's first action was to buy a rugged four-wheel drive truck that could climb the slopes. Most of his travel was in his horse's saddle. There were wild steers from a previous renter to find, fences to fix and cows and bulls to buy. They were located forty-five miles up the often one-lane road from Livermore and two miles back into the ranch from the road. They had no phone. We saw her once a month when she came to town to shop for groceries.

The first Easter they were there, Jacquie and I helped Karen fence a small playpen in the grass outside the kitchen window for their daughter, Melani. The fencing was hail screen to keep any rattlesnakes out of the play area. They saw a mountain lion and knew wild pigs were present on the ranch. "Don, it was the last day of August that the crisis occurred, remember?"

"Yes. I still have the Labor Day Mercury Newspaper that proclaimed in large, bold type, **TOT RESCUED FROM MT. TOP**. It started much as all accidents do. Karen had taken the garbage basket from under the sink to the outside trash burner. She didn't get the cabinet door completely closed and her toddler daughter, Melani, nicknamed Mel, went to investigate. When Karen returned, Mel was licking an ant poison container she had found in the cabinet.

Darrel was out somewhere on his horse, so Karen put Mel into the truck and started for the road. There was a house near the road that a family occupied on weekends, The first of September was a weekday this year, and no one would be home. She was mistaken. One son, a sheriff's deputy, had come up to the house for the day. He immediately pulled out his radio and called for rescue. Putting the women into his squad car he soon navigated the twelve miles to the top of Mt. Hamilton to meet a helicopter on a road switch-back. The pilot quickly put Karen and Mel on top of a hospital where Mel's stomach was pumped with no ill effects.

"Their lives have remained interesting Don. After the ranch was sold they moved to town where he managed a land bank before buying a ranch and building a home in the pass. Now he has another ranch job as the financial employee for an outfit with holdings in several states. He didn't need a four-wheel truck for this: he bought part interest in an airplane."

"I don't know if you picked it up Self, but their son Eric, is planning on building a house near his folks. He is a warehouse manager here in town and his wife, Michele is the firm's office manager."

"Yeah. They too seem just as busy and involved as his parents so you and JJL don't get to see them or your great grandson Blake much even though they work only three miles from you."

Chapter 14

Relax While You Can, Don
How Do You Plan for What's Ahead?

Two weeks later the default setting of my internal alarm awakens me. I dress, and after feeding the cats, fix my coffee. As I enjoy the brew, Mocha arrives on her penthouse roof and our quality time begins another day with satisfaction for both of us. I have time to enjoy my word processor for an hour or so. I need a break. After I put on my shoes and don my white walking hat, I step outside. The morning air smells fantastic as my lungs pick up its freshness. It will be an outstanding day with this quality. An adult in a car is throwing rolled papers onto the driveways while driving alternately on both sides of the street. The first of the dog owners are beginning to exercise themselves and their charges. As the dawn brightens, I meet singles out jogging and couples walking. Most of the folks out at this time are in the Junes through Augusts of their lives.

Turning the corner to the south, I notice four robins breakfast-searching on a neighbor's lawn. They run four or five steps, and upon stopping, cock their heads to one side and appear to listen to the earth. Suddenly they stab the lawn and come up with a small worm. Do they hunt with their ears, their eyes or both? Since I don't have a lawn or plants with berries, robins don't visit me, and I enjoy these bright-breasted fellows for a moment.

The high wires two blocks to the east seem to be a gathering spot for blue jays and doves. Stepping along the sidewalk of a park, I enjoy watching the dozen crows that are now doing their exercise bit as they, also, search for breakfast. Some are holding small acorns with one foot while they crack them with their strong beaks. Others have found a French fry from a soccer game last night and are bickering over it. One large jet-black bird walks at a deliberate pace with head held high. Crows are reported to be one of the smartest birds we see.

A squirrel runs across the street just as a large white dog comes around the corner. Spotting the squirrel, the dog gives chase. Three feet ahead of the dog, the squirrel approaches a power pole but it does not jump straight onto the pole as I expect. That move would have ended with the dog jumping and capturing it. Instead, the squirrel goes past the pole, U-turns and then scampers up the backside of the pole. The dog, mouth open to grasp the squirrel, doesn't see the squirrel's hidden U-turn and runs past the pole. It is a very confused dog that stops and looks around for the prey it almost captured. It is easy to read the canine's reaction: "I don't believe it! That fellow just disappeared. A magic squirrel!"

I see that we are losing some neighbors. The "For Sale" sign is up in their front yard. We have enjoyed watching them raise their sons, and we think alike on many things. Although we did not socialize, as he is allergic to cats, and JJL doesn't venture out to other homes, we will miss them. I wonder who our new neighbors will be. Will they be young and keep to themselves? Will an investor buy the house and rent it to a group of five boys, as happened to the house across from Rosie? Our quiet, stable neighborhood will change a bit. I need to act my part as a good neighbor. The story is told of a fellow who moved into a new farm neighborhood and asked the first farmer he saw, "Are the neighbors good here?"

"What were they like where you came from?"

"Great."

"You'll find the same kind here, but if you had answered, Not good, I would have answered, 'Not good here also.'

Believing I control a lot of my own destiny, I will be a good neighbor.

Today's walk is ending, and I can see our house. The morning is now as light as it will be until the thin layer of fog burns off and the sun has the sky to itself. I make the final turn and come up our walkway. I should design a flying ramp to eliminate the two shallow steps if we need to use the wheelchair more. A flying ramp over the little streambed, which our bridge spans, would complement the house exterior. I can design it but I doubt if I have the energy to form and pour it.

I enter the house, and as I head for the red chair, I notice a picture is askew on the wall near JJL's recliner. I heard a little noise as I turned off the TV last night. Jacquie must have fallen against the wall as she was stepping into her walker. I was facing the opposite way as I reached for the switch, and she didn't say anything. It must be depressing to sense you are losing control and not know what to do about your problem.

I begin reviewing the tasks of the day. One chore is to go to the watercolor association gallery to pick up my paintings from a past show. There is a requirement that participating artists spend two afternoons minding the gallery. If we get a caregiver for JJL, I will enter the next show and hope to get into it. Painting and art are an activities I enjoy. I have written a manuscript on how to physically check a house before buying it. I need to illustrate the text, and that will be a welcome challenge. Inserting drawings into the text I understand; adding photos is a skill I must learn.

Sometime today I will fill out a health care directive for emergencies for each of us. It's been a long time since we prepared an Advanced Health Care Form advising the medical team what to do in an extreme emergency. I took my present directive with me twice to a cardiac unit where I was to have invasive procedures done, and had to explain it to my advantage. It had the correct wording and message, but the lawyer goofed in its format. "Please revive me," it said in a paragraph. Exceptions, - if I will always be a vegetable, cannot recover, and several other conditions were listed below the paragraph, bulleted with dark black spots. The doctor looking at the document did as we all do. He skipped the paragraph and saw only the bullets. He said, "Are you sure you don't want to be revived if something goes wrong?"

"Read the paragraph above the bullets," I direct.

"Oh, there is a difference," he replies after a few seconds of reading.

As a caregiver, I must plan some refreshing times for myself or I may burn out, a common occurrence I hear. I enjoy my morning walk and my quality times with Mocha, but I should also consider fishing with my son and grandson and make plans to continue judging art shows and painting. If I don't maintain or expand my interests, I may suffer from a lack of interaction with others- either by choice, like JJL, or because isolation is imposed on me like my neighbor, Rosie. The book by Jimmy Carter, *The Virtues of Aging,* Karen gave me at Christmas is written along those lines. He says rather than to let-up at retirement, expand everything intellectually, socially and health-wise. If you've always wanted to learn a foreign language, chess or computers, now is the time. Launch out into social interactions and adopt an exercise program. I remember a Rabbi writing on the Internet, "Heaven is a good life lived, and if there is more after that, so much the better!" I guess he is saying we are the captains of our destiny, so be a good captain and choose fine navigation.

"Don't forget," Self reminds me. "Plan on JJL's doctor's appointments the next two Mondays, and the one with the insurance nurse tomorrow." This nurse will fill out a questionnaire necessary to start home health care from a policy we initiated several years ago. I will soon have some help with JJL's care giving. I've done well so far in caring for her in spite of two different doctors at the ER suggesting we should consider a rest home placement for JJL. If having Jane, our once a week housekeeper, help us two afternoons a week isn't enough, our insurance will provide for rest home placement.

As I think of these health items, I remember the results of my blood tests I received yesterday. They were within the normal ranges. Either my cooking or my behavior is rewarding me. Self laughs and whispers, "The results are in spite of your cooking." He's getting testy as he ages.

I rest a few minutes and it's time to feed the cats and the birds. Soon it will be time to awaken Jacquie for her breakfast. "Things are back to normal," I think as I reach for a new can of cat food. "Our episodes with the HMO are past." How wrong I am! The episodes will just get more complicated and frightening.

Chapter 15

"911 and 911 Again!"
Togetherness on 580 and 680

It is an interesting evening of TV. We watch the eleven o'clock news with no warning of the adventures to unfold in the wee hours ahead, or the strangers that we will meet after going to bed. We don't snack, and I soon have JJL undressed and ready for bed. As I turn down the bed coverings Mocha joins us, as bed making or bed changing falls into her job description. She mews softly as she cavorts and rolls about, communicating with us. She always wants to be near.. She may be somewhere else, but when she hears our voices, she comes in a dash to join us.

It takes me only a moment to join Jacquie in bed as she turns off the bedside light.

"How are the shoulders, Don? Still ache?"

"They still do, but it's also in the chest. I took several aspirins, and I hope they work soon so I can get to sleep."

They don't work, and in time the pain is bad enough to get me out of bed. I take a nitroglycerin tablet in case it is a heart pain, and go to the red rocker. After five minutes, I take a second nitro, and it also does not provide relief. I've wanted to toss the tablets in the little nitro carrier I always carry and fill it with fresh pills. The tiny tablets are viable for three months, and that time is up. I break the seal on a new bottle and take a potent tablet, thinking, "How can these little pills, half the size of a match head, do enough good to save a man's life?"

"You'd better call for some advice, Don," my now awake Self admonishes.

I call the HMO advice nurse. "I have a pain in my chest, and I wonder if it is bad enough to come the ER?"

"Tell me about it, how bad it is and when it started."

I do the explanations and tell her my by-pass surgery was only two or three years ago.

"Come to the ER," she tells me.

"I shouldn't drive that far. If I had a heart attack and crossed the road, I might kill someone else," I reason aloud. "My wife is not driving. The state has revoked her license."

"Call 911 and come in. Any chest pain should be taken seriously."

"You sound like a wife," I reply, a standard quip to someone giving orders.

"I mean it, and now," she says and hangs up. End of argument. No recourse! No one on the line to argue with. She wins, period.

I call 911, and after giving them the address I tell them, "Please do not use the lights and sirens, or I will bolt the door and not let you in."

I dress JJL, unlock the door and turn on the porch light. It is only a matter of minutes before I hear a large truck grumble around the corner and start up the hill. This new hook-and-ladder truck with bright rotating light parks in the middle of the street; it appears to be as long as our lot is wide. As four firemen in full yellow fire-fighting garb come into the house, Mocha streaks into the bedroom and under the bed. The fireman's division of labor is automatic and a joy to watch. While one kneels and opens a box of emergency gear, another breaks out a stethoscope to listen to my chest and then questions me about what has happened. A third snaps a finger clamp on me to check the oxygen level of my blood and gives me a spray of nitroglycerin under the tongue. Someone has the blood pressure cuff on my arm while the fourth is acting like a court reporter with a clipboard. He records my every answer and adds questions of his own. There is no casual conversation. They are all business. My eye, sharpened by my many years of being a school principal, house inspector, and an artist tells me this is indeed a skilled group.

An ambulance arrives. The attendants come through the open door, and are immediately a part of the team. They take over the site responsibility, and the information already gathered is given them. They need to listen with their own stethoscope before snapping a gurney into its carrying position. A moment later I am on the gurney and my trip is ready to begin, or so I think.

"Where's my wife?" I ask. "Can she ride in the cab? She is forbidden to drive, and she cannot stay alone as she falls."

"She's in the bathroom," a fireman replies, and then it happens. There is a loud thump from the far side of the dining room.

"She's fallen!" one of the team reports, and part of my team leaves to kneel and check on her. The report continues, "She fell against the table and cut her head on the way down. She's out. Call a backup ambulance." While one or two work with her, an EMT goes to his unit to get a carrying board to transport her.

By the time my remaining crewmembers finish strapping me down for transport the other fellows have taken her vital signs and strapped her to the carrying board. She is ready for the second unit, which is now arriving and adding its flashing red lights to those of the others. Our street is full of emergency vehicles, and we have eight men in a house that seldom has more than two people.

As we start for the door, I ask a fireman to check that the cat pan by the garage door has water, as we might not be back soon. "It's not here," he calls. Then he finds it on the counter.

"JJL's having memory problems again," Self tells me.

"You're right. The cats are important to her, so she went to fill the pan and forgot what she was doing partway through the process."

We are out the door. As I am placed into the ambulance, the fire truck goes up the hill and is gone. Our exit from the neighborhood becomes confused and prolonged. I wonder why we don't make a U-turn and come back down Lincoln Avenue, but I'm not driving this trip, and I have no experience being a back seat driver while looking out a rear-facing window into darkness. Soon I sense we have stopped, are backing and making a U-turn in a dead-end street. In a few minutes we repeat the process in yet another court. The driver is lost. Finally we roll out of town and through the night on the all but deserted freeways. "You'd better be thankful you're not having a full blown attack," Self confides with me. "Your luck is holding."

"I know about you," the attendant at the ER admitting counter tells me as I'm wheeled past her. "Your wife is here and she talked."

"I'm glad she made it. Her driver didn't get lost like mine did. Is there a rental break on a double room?"

"Nope! She is in Emergency room B and you're going into A, which has the kind of equipment doctors need to monitor your heart." The lady is all business and she turns to her next task. She knows how to deal with smart alecs like me. Ignore them and get on with it!

As I am placed onto the bed, a nurse reaches for the EKG sensor cups and tears the tabs off their sticky surfaces. "Why don't aging men go bald on the chest instead of the head? Removing those things would be much less painful. I wish I had used the few minutes before the firemen arrived to shave my chest."

"Just lean back and we'll get a blood draw next." This lady too is all business and she too ignores me. Good!

"I know," I say, "and your Dracula who gathers blood doesn't hurt as much as the removal of these sticky cups. He's very good at drawing blood I found when I was here before. I hope he's here this morning. By the way, can you find out how my wife, Jacquie, is doing? Please? She's probably in unit B." I know from past experience I will be here six hours at a minimum before a second blood draw can tell if certain chemicals have been released into the blood, signaling a heart attack.

Seven hours pass without incident to me other than my worry about my Jacquie. The firemen did report blood on her forehead, but a hospital worker relays she is doing fine.

"Knowing she is OK will help you, Don," Self assures me. It sounds as if he said that with compassion.

It is then I have a surprising sight. A gurney containing a lady patient has been wheeled into the center and stopped outside my door. If they asked her to use a bedpan there she would have been insulted. However, her catheter is emptied in plain sight without anyone, including her, noticing or minding. So much for the sense of modesty!

"You didn't have a heart attack," the doctor informs me as if he is as relieved as I am. "You can get up after signing some paperwork and go to your wife. I hear she doesn't have major problems."

The early morning crew in her part of the ward looks familiar, since we had been in this unit on the same shift two weeks ago. JJL is still having bouts of dizziness, but she is about to be released. The doctor's answer to my questions about the condition of dizziness is one we will remember. "Try this prescription." It is a travel sickness remedy. "If that doesn't help, check her into a rest home." That is a pretty straightforward message delivered without any preliminaries.

I agree with Self's appraisal, "That was out of the blue. I'll bet he flunked the med school's bedside manners course."

The pharmacy gives us the over-the-counter form of the medicine. We find it inexpensive, and it helps to a certain extent, at least enough to keep JJL out of a rest home for now. Will her condition change? If so, which way and when? No one seems to know.

Karen and Darrel are out of the state so I phone Jon just as he and his family are to leave for the mountains for a week. "Yes, I can come and bring you home," he says. "What are you doing at the hospital again?"

"It's a long story. We're OK. We'll meet you in the emergency parking lot."

We are both fine, except JJL has a very black eye where she fell against the table. Unfortunately, it is the eye that had the cancer surgery a week before.

It is time to go home and try to catch the sleep we have missed. We were lucky last night, and also thankful for the excellent help that came to assist us. How much longer will this continue, I wonder?

"If it's not going to get better, will it get worse?" Self whispers. He shares my worries.

We find the cats weathered the night of flashing lights and strange men. Latte is on the bed where she and Jacquie will be taking an afternoon nap. She wakens to look at us and opens her mouth in a typical cat yawn.

As I help JJL change her clothes and get her to bed I find a variety of bruises and even fingermarks on her shoulder blades where the 911 team placed their hands to lift her to the transport pad. I go to the fire station the next day to thank the crew that took care of us and to ask if JJL was unconscious when they went to her. I am wondering if she fell because she was dizzy, or if she became unconscious first and then fell. "That was a fill-in crew last night. One is now in the Sierras fighting a forest fire and others are either off-duty or at other stations. They said she was unconscious when we came on duty this morning."

"That doesn't answer your question, Don. Did she faint and fall or get dizzy and knock herself out as she hit the table?" Self and I could make a good team.

The situations are over, I tell myself. This time we will be back to routines again for awhile. Again, I am wrong. My pain will return in two weeks, and I will have a big dose of bad luck with an overly helpful advice nurse.

"You can't win 'em all, Don."

"Yeah, but I'd like to up my batting average. Real bad!"

Chapter 16

She Listens With Her Mouth!
I Just Miss the ER Room

Today's a bad day. It starts that way. I waken and dress before dawn. I have a small but persistent pain at the center of the lower ribs. The pain is not as severe as the one that caused an ambulance trip two weeks ago. I think it is the result of stress.

Just in case today's pain is heart related, I take a nitroglycerin tablet and soon afterward, two aspirins, in case it is something else. The aspirins will not hurt me. I remember the firemen gave me two baby aspirins, together with a spray of nitro under the tongue. My next action is to make a cup of hot tea and find my way in the growing light to Grandma's old red rocker. Here I will monitor the pain and contemplate my next action.

The pain eases. I retrieve the HMO member medical guidebook from the shelf and turn to the chest pain page. As I start to read, Mocha arrives on my lap and begs for some petting. Petting while reading can be difficult and it becomes almost impossible when the end of a long bushy tail rubs across your face repeatedly. I found angina is a problem of blood supply to the heart muscle, and a heart attack is a similar but a worse condition of blood supply. The book suggests that the two conditions differ by being either less than, or more than, twenty minutes in duration. I don't know how long the pain had been present before I awakened. The explanation in the book didn't seem to be definitive. Anxiety is not mentioned.

Has the pain lasted more or less than twenty minutes? It isn't as bad as two weeks ago, is it? I try the one-to-ten pain scale doctors use, but I can't remember the reading two weeks ago. I don't think it is heart problem, but I'm not a doctor. I wonder if it is really stress again. I take my stress medicine. I had stopped taking it before the other attack. So is it stress, or isn't it? How does stress chest pain differ from angina or heart pain, which can be manifested in many ways, further confusing a sufferer? Is there really a stress chest pain? I call the HMO advice nurse and ask her how the two differ. "How does a stress pain feel?" I asked.

"I have your history on my computer screen, and you have a history of angina," is her answer.

"They didn't use that word two weeks ago when I was in the ER room," I reply.

"Why do you ask about stress?" she counters.

To give her the reason I start to say, "My wife and I …"

I get no further. "Are you calling about yourself or your wife? She demands to know.

Thinking I can't be interrupted if I only use one word, I tell her, "Both."

"I don't have her profile on the computer," my advisor informs me. "I can deal with only one patient at a time." I can't get an opportunity to say that my wife is having severe health problems, putting stress on me as a spouse and chief caregiver. "Is the pain worse now?" she asks. I think your listening skills are making it much worse, I say to myself. "I can't make determinations," she tells me. "'I'll talk to the advice doctor on duty. I'll be back." I'm afraid she will be.

After a long period of time she does come back to say, "I am booking an appointment with your doctor."

My cell phone slips from my ear, cutting me off. I have no way to know which nurse she is for a call to apologize. I'll bet she is shaking her head about what a problem person I am.

I wish I hadn't made the call. That lady was a contrast to good communicators. She didn't let me finish sentences. She listened with her mouth.

"So what?" Self says - "She is a turkey with a nurse's badge."

The next day my morning starts much, much better. I have no chest pain. Over coffee in the red chair, with Mocha beside me, I consider a number of things. I need to take better control of parts of my life. The first change is a longer walk. The over-the-counter pills I take on the advice of my daughter-in-law, Karen, seem to be helping me grow more replacement knee cartilage. I can walk again with no pain. I will take my three-mile walk to Safeway and back. I cut through the side yard of a vacant house and follow truck tracks across a plowed field.

Since a super hardware store and its parking lot are being built I can no longer cut across a different field that used to be my route. The ground squirrels and the weeds have been bulldozed, and the area is fenced from trespassers.

On the way home with a small bag of groceries hanging from each wrist, I step from beside the vacant house onto Colgate Way where I meet two ladies half my age who are faithful walkers. Over the months I have learned to appreciate these pleasant women. I can't remember their names, so I'll call the tall one who is recovering from a gall bladder operation Jake. She reminds me of the proverbial Jake, the tall country boy of folklore with a perpetual smile, only hers is a grin instead of a smile. Her eyes never stop smiling. Jake says, "Hi! How ya been?"

"OK, I guess."

"What d'ya mean, you guess? You been under the weather?"

"No, I had a pain problem yesterday morning that worried me."

"Didn't you call an advice nurse?" the other lady asks. "Those people were very helpful to me two years ago when my husband was dying."

"I did, and I wished I hadn't," I reply.

"How come?" Jake asks. "No help?"

"That woman listened with her mouth. I couldn't finish a sentence without her interrupting. I wanted to know the difference between stress and heart pains."

I describe the frustrating phone call, and conclude, "The uncertainty of Jacquie's health, the slowness of communication from the insurance company and my tiredness from care-giving is probably my problem. I need to learn to live with problems."

"Were you OK the rest of the day?" Jake's companion wants to know.

"Yes, it was a great day. I didn't have my question answered, but I will talk to the doctor. I've booked an appointment with Dr. Watson, the head doctor, or should I say doctor of heads? She's a psychologist with a less intimidating title. She knows my wife and me, and we have a lot of confidence in her. I think one of her best strengths is the ability to listen with her ears and to get to the heart of the concerns."

By then we walkers have turned down Lincoln Avenue. I wave goodbye to my nameless friends as I head up my walkway.

Sitting down after putting the groceries away, I am greeted by Mocha. I have returned from my walk across the open field with a variety of interesting odors that have hitchhiked on my shoes. She is fascinated with the stories they tell. It is time for the red chair, a cup of tea and some reflecting. She jumps into the chair seat beside me and puts her hips beside mine. She begins to tell me she loves me with several choruses of purring, loud enough for my hearing aids to receive her message. When it comes to relieving stress, one Mocha is worth dozens of nurses like the one yesterday.

I remember someone saying, "The Golden Years are a pathway of lead bricks spray-painted gold." I hope the bricks in my walkway into the future are solid regardless of color. I didn't want problems in the trek ahead. Boy! Do I have surprises before I take too many more steps!

Chapter 17

Valves, Dizziness and Drizzles
Why Should I Live So Long?

It's early morning, At my age I am always glad to welcome another day. I work at the word processor until my eyes become bleary. Then it's time to take a break. I put the computer to sleep, as I'll be off on my predawn walk. Latte comes to sit beside me in the conversation pit and watches me put on my shoes. I wonder how many times I've put on shoes. Seventy-five years times 365 days plus putting on overshoes several times a day minus the days I went barefoot plus the times I had to change from work shoes to dress shoes. Ah forget it!

The walk is starting fine. A few mockingbirds are singing and several people are out walking. Younger ladies have their dogs along, or they stroll in pairs, enjoying each other's company while exercising. I call to one young lady with a big dog, "You'll have to walk faster to wear that big guy down."

"You've got that right," she replies as they turn to go down another street.

"Fifty years ago Californians were a lot skinnier than the folks we left in Kansas but that has changed," Self reminds me.

"Dad always said, 'We grow the food so we should eat well. If there's any left over, we can sell to others.' "He also said, when he saw a thin woman," 'Her man didn't feed her very well!' and he meant it."

Now, there seems to be a correlation to the number of fast food establishments available and our body size. Changes in our way of life allow the grocer to stock many more instant meals which are high in what we don't need. A study finds our lessening amount of sleep is also leading to obesity. I'd better use my sleeping pills when I waken in the night, I tell myself.

Arriving at the railroad overpass I stride upward until I can see the hills rimming our valley. They are just beginning to show against the lightening sky. The stars are starting to use their dimmer switches

For the last ten days, I've been so tired that I just sat much of the time. I didn't even want to read or play solitaire at the computer. That's not my style. I want to jog right up to my funeral. I want to drive up to the Pearly Gates and hand in my keys. No wheelchairs or death sledges for me. I think it's the medication to relax my nerves and make me easier to live with that's causing the problem. Jacquie doesn't have this problem as severe as I do, so I think I'll ask to be put on her medication.

On the way home I am thankful Safeway had a nice bathroom for me to use a few minutes ago. We can get new heart valves, eye corneas, artificial ears and have valve seats reworked on our house plumbing. So why can't we get new or rebuilt elimination valves for our bodies?

When I asked a doctor that question he replied, "It's a low priority item in the medical field. We use a catheter instead." I realize Wal Marts and grocery stores can sell panty liners and disposable panties to solve the immediate problem. I guess that is an improvement over the cloth diapers Dad and Mom had to use for Grandpa Andy's colon leakage.

His lack of bladder control was solved when Grandpa's doctor inserted a catheter for several weeks. After insertion, a few puffs of air inflated a marble-sized balloon in the bladder to keep the catheter from slipping out. One day the balloon would not deflate and couldn't be removed. The doctor looked at Dad and said, "'Guess I'll have to break the balloon to get it out." A few squeezes of the air syringe and there was a small, audible pop.

Grandpa jumped and asked, "V'ot's 'dat?" It worked. The deflated unit slid out and a new catheter was soon in place.

Grandpa was lucky, the folks gave him good care through his eighties and into his nineties. Now families are scattered and there is no one at home to care for the elderly, as everyone has to work to afford the lifestyle they choose. So it's off to the rest home and oftentimes, questionable care. As our population lives longer, societies need to find ways to care for the elderly increases. "Self, I've said it before I'm sure, but up till WW II, people cared for their parents at home. When I was a boy I had a grandparent living with us, as did my friends. We knew about aging. After the war the women did not come home to care for parents. They went to work elsewhere and the rest home industry was born. Their children, the Baby Boomers, now don't understand the parent's aging problems nor do they know what's ahead for themselves."

"Market tip," Self announces. "Invest in rest and care homes." Scientists are working to extend our lifetimes and we assume this is desirable. "Don," Self continues, "if you live to be a hundred twenty five, you could be living with your kids, who would be a hundred years of age. Even if you lived with your grandchildren, they would be seventy, hardly in the best of shape to take on substantial care."

This kind of situation would affect the quality of life for everyone. How old is old enough? I pose a related question to Self; "Do we all have go to midnight, December thirty-one?"

Another factor is the increased cost of living longer. Seniors now have large pharmaceutical costs. Self offers another market tip: "Buy pharmaceuticals." The need for pills for seniors will continue for many more years. I can imagine the health insurance premiums! The heavy costs of major medical procedures will also continue. Once a bypass operation was a rarity. Now, many individuals are having a second one, and even a third. My quadruple bypass operation was reported to cost $70,000, but that amount would be much higher now. Funding insurance and HMOs for the increased costs will take an increased amount out of the take-home checks.

Arriving home after my walk I go past the foot of our bed. JJL is still asleep. I decide to take a bimonthly newspaper with me to the bathroom. Guess what is advertised on the back page? "If you are older and have bladder problems, leaks, surprises, you need to order our pills with cranberry extract, they work!" The paper caters to older citizens and zeros in on our problems. That's good marketing. I don't need more pills, though. It now takes me an hour a week to count and place our weekly supply into the correct daily doses.

The cats arrive in our bathroom and receive petting before I stand and pull the zipper. Men becoming seniors learn that standing and aiming is no longer a sure thing. Unlike the little boys just learning to point and go, we have learned the trigonometry of aiming. However, in both cases, there is not much to aim. We old fellows suffer from one other problem – a lack of muzzle velocity.

I saw a set of absorbent panties advertised on TV this week. I started to giggle but had second thoughts. "I don't have to use them as an Octoberian. Hallelujah. But perhaps my time is coming as I enter another decade of being an old man.

JJL is having good week. She is using the walker the HMO gave her two months ago. We are again walking to the corner and back. She has shown no odd thought processes lately; however, she collapsed four times in three days. The HMO has an extension service, so a physiotherapist, a nurse trained to monitor medications and a home nurse came to check on her. The home nurse arrived first and checked JJL's vitals and found them to be as they should be. Then the medical nurse went over the medicines we have and our charts on dosage and frequency. There are no physical impediments in the house, but it is suggested we use a chair in the shower to prevent falls and a showerhead on a hose. Each nurse thought Jacquie is doing well and discharges herself from further service.

Are we now over her hump of ill health? I hope so. Is it all sunlight ahead now that her clouds are lifting? The cats are giving her renewed attention, which is like the silver lining of any cloud. She doesn't want to talk about her falls but wants to sit and sleep or watch TV.

I'm too positive. Squalls are headed her way with a vengeance. One afternoon while walking behind her walker I notice she slows and begins to falter. I am close enough to catch her as she starts to fall backward. She is rigid, not bending at the waist. She relaxes momentarily and is unconscious for a few seconds. As she revives I get her to bed. By then she is fully alert.

Later, I awaken in the middle of the night with her calling, "Don. Don!" I start looking for her in the darkened house with no success. At first, I do not look in the right area. As I come into the kitchen, she whispers loudly, "I'm here on the floor." Just as I arrive, I feel something give under my bare foot two feet before her head. I find I have stepped upon her glasses and popped the lenses from the frame. But luck is with us. I did not break the lenses or cut my foot.

I want to ask, "What are you doing down there?" but she saves me the trouble.

"I had a headache and came out for a towel and some ice. I got dizzy and fell."

"Why didn't you awaken me? It's my job to run errands for you until you're one hundred percent."

"You do so much for me and I didn't want to awaken you."

"Isn't that is a statement of love and appreciation?" Self whispers to me in his half sleep.

"You chose a good spot to fall backward out of the walker. I don't know how you were lucky enough to fall in the passageway between the stove and the counter. How's your head? Did you crack it on the floor? You should have fallen a step sooner so you would have hit carpet instead the hard kitchen vinyl."

"It hurts. You'll have to help me up, Don!"

I struggle to get her on her feet. She's of little help, and all but dead weight. "After I get you back to bed I'll get an ice pack for your head."

"Oh please! It is hurting so bad I don't feel the headache I was trying to lessen." While the head will be tender for a day of so, she is to suffer from a sore posterior for better than a week. Each day she will reposition herself often as she sits and watches TV.

Early one morning I'm told, "Oh, Don, I don't feel good. I'm so dizzy. You'd better walk beside me as I get up and head for the recliner, but first, I'd better sit there for awhile." I need to be present even though she has a walker as she forgets to use it. In time I will find that she can black out while using the walker and then fall. She does not get better.

"I'll call the advice nurse."

"No. They'll want me to come to the ER."

"Great! They need to see you while you're having an attack. Maybe we can get some resolution if they see you in action." I call the advice nurse and after a quick consultation with an advice doctor she instructs us to come to the ER facility. It is a nice predawn ride, even with the early commuters.

The visit does not result in any new conclusion and she is sent home. She's soon back in her recliner. I take her a small chocolate-filled cookie, low enough in sugar content for her diabetic condition. The odor of the chocolate awakens Mocha and she arrives on my wife's lap to investigate. She makes an appearance whenever a wrapper is opened. Chocolate is poison to cats, so she will have to suffer without a treat.

This business of becoming ready for elder years is like getting ready for a hard winter in the cold country. Planning ahead is necessary. Like the fact that there is less light in winter, I find I am having less energy in my October years. Reading my thoughts, Self sighs, "Another fact the Baby Boomers will learn by surprise, I'll bet."

Now that we are home again I believe JJL is feeling better. Instead of asking me what I'm fixing for dinner she arrives in the kitchen and wants to take over. She has forgotten that she needs assistance and arrives without the walker. However, it must be said she varies like the month of November, one bright day followed by one or more dismal ones.

I need to prepare the shower for safer bathing. Since she doesn't think she can get out of our tub, she uses the shower exclusively. Two years ago I installed two grab bars in the shower for her. We have been showering together for a year so ever since JJL started having her dizzy spells. Fortunately, when we built the house three decades ago we chose a shower pan five feet long rather than the small ones more commonly installed then. I stand behind her with arms around her while she shampoos and bathes. The shower is long enough for me to squat and wash her legs while she hangs onto the railings with both hands.

I have worried I might not be able to hold her soapy body if she falls. The HMO's nurse recommended a chair and an extension hose. A few minutes shopping and a few more to install them I think. Am I wrong! The shower hose is easy to find, but finding a lawn chair in mid-October is another matter. The chairs are sold out or have been returned to inventory. When in doubt, where does one go? To a drug store. There is where I find the chair. When I was a kid the only things a drugstore offered was drugs and a soda fountain. "Another thing the Boomers don't know is that the fountain had a variety of flavors for colas," my invisible companion whispers. "There were chocolate, vanilla, pineapple, strawberry, and cherry colas. Remember?"

"Yeah. Cherry colas were a favorite of mine. Jacquie liked chocolate ones on our dates."

The nineteen dollar showerhead has only four shower patterns but that is OK with JJL. More important, it is small in size and she can hold it. The chair occupies one third of the floor space. Even so, that will become a problem.

We try a shower after running water at the nearby sink until it is warm. I reach into the shower and open the valve, a big mistake. The showerhead on the end of the hose is on the floor and is not stable. It swings around the shower floor in jet-propelled circles, spraying water out the open door and hits the cats who are in a curiosity mode outside. It might have been funny in a cartoon, but neither the cats nor JJL find it amusing. I reach in, grab the hose and adjust the flow.

I shower the plastic chair for awhile to warm it as sitting naked on a cold plastic chair could ruin her shower. She opens the sliding door then and complains, "Some water is coming out onto the floor." It is evident more adjustments are necessary. I really want to say it wasn't getting to the floor before you opened the door but I have second thoughts. I understand being the head of the household is only a figurehead.

It is time to start showering. She starts to lower herself to sit onto an almost warm chair and I stand behind her. There are only eight inches between my bare bottom and the cold tile behind me. She starts to lose her balance but I catch her. The more quickly I get her into the chair the better. The trouble is her heading into the shower rather than backing into it. I have to turn her around before I can bend her into the chair. "We have a way to go," I tell her. The first lesson the next time will center on entering the shower."

Then she stands up and asks; "Do you want to shower first?"

"No. If I shower first and get clean then your dirty water will splash onto me!" I think about my statement and decide I have said enough. Things aren't too bad yet. My bathing goes fairly well after I manage to hold the showerhead to keep it from hitting her while I use both hands to open the shampoo bottle.

Handing the showerhead to her I announce, "It's your turn."

"Not so hard. Turn it down, Don! My gosh, how can you stand it spraying so hard?" How can I reach the control, which is in front of her? I manage to ease the flow and decide she is not going to have a shower. She is going to have a drizzle. "Hand me the shampoo please. Soap my back." All is going well until it is time to wash her legs and feet. There isn't room for me to bend over in the chair or kneel to do that. Also, how can I wash her bottom when she is sitting on it? She stands up and not only does she get her bottom washed she gets dirty water on me. Again, prudence and better than a half century of matrimonial experience keep my mouth closed but my head is shaking behind hers. "I'm ready to have my back and legs dried, Don."

The drizzle is over but the exit from the shower remains. If there is to be a fall I can hear me calling 911: "Help me get my wife out of the drizzle."

I leave the shower stall and reach back in to help her. "Come out here. I'll help you."

"Is there room for me to walk between the toilet, you and the shower?"

"Yes." She does and I have a towel on the floor for her to step onto to avoid slipping. There is soon room for me to do all of the necessary drying. "We have to think this process through before you drizzle again," I tell her. "With the chair outside you could step into the shower and hold onto the bars while I place the chair inside."

"Yes, but it would be cold without a warming! You would have to warm it first. I notice several personal pronouns directed my way.

"Maybe I should put seat belts on the chair like those on your wheelchair." Somehow drizzling with her isn't as exciting as showering with her was a half century ago.

The cats are waiting for us outside the shower. When JJL goes to the bathroom, Latte and Mocha follow. That's just like country school years ago, I think. When one girl went to the outhouse, they all went!

I slip a dress over JJL's shoulders and help her to the recliner. It is then Self makes an appearance to ask, "Are you OK, Don? Relax. Remember stress and worry caused you a 911 call just a short while back." I take his input seriously. I won't be any good to JJL if I get down. I wonder if we'll be drizzling two weeks from now or if I'll need to wash her in bed with a washcloth.

I decide follow up on my earlier call to the insurance company about some part time help. I need to have some short breaks. When they say OK, can I find any help?

Chapter 18

My October Sky Rockets
Wet Noise

Have your rockets or plans ever misfired? Jacquie and I suffered several misfires with our ground fireworks this week. One left us laughing and changing the bed, while the shower solution remains unsolved. But first, let me explain why I use the metaphor of fireworks to lead into these latest incidents.

Through our July and August of life, our thoughts are often on September and October, the retirement and golden years. We expect fun and excitement to rise and burst like huge colorful rockets, with excitement and delights for all. I can't say this has been true for me in the latter weeks of my October of life. I will say I have managed to shoot off a lot of small ground fireworks most of my life and enjoy the excitement I create. Any large rockets I've sent are bursting, and what I'm seeing is a lot of little sparkles. While colorful, they do not generate a lot of Oohs and Aaahs.

As we shut down the working shift and bring the tools home for the last time, we dream of what September and October will be like. "You think you can get up whenever you want like all seniors tell themselves," Self giggles. "You can retire the alarm clock and put it on a pension, you vow."

We can take classes in Tropical Rain Forest Walking in Hawaii or Brazil, or study the whales from a cruise ship. We might consider having a six-wheel land cruiser and to go exploring back roads in other states. Perhaps a graduate class in Probability in Las Vegas would be interesting.

JJL and I didn't get that far in October. In our late August or early September we did send up two rockets, a flight to Scotland and another to Spain. We also discovered the two Fs of buffets on Sundays: Fun and Fat. Going to a Sunday buffet is now one of the small ground rockets we fire every six weeks or so. We used to go more often, but because somehow calories seem to count faster at this stage of life, we now put more time between buffet trips to slow down our weight accumulation. Sometimes the brunch offerings can be a problem. JJL has developed a dislike for several of foods she's not allergic to. Being diabetic is another problem. It's too bad she hasn't picked up a dislike for chocolate, pie, and frappe. On the other hand, she has few pleasures so I guess it's chocolate and other desserts in minute quantities.

We do enjoy sparklers and a pinwheel now and then. My junior college writing class is a highlight for me each week. I hope to expand my interest in the Internet as well. Perhaps our greatest daily enjoyment is the great companionship and enjoyment we receive from our coffee cats: Latte and Mocha. Not only do we enjoy them, I know they have had a significant effect on JJL's health. The cats love to be petted and seem to enjoy our company. "And I notice both you and JJL love to stroke your felines. Like the cats, both of you wear a smile. It's a two way street Don." Self is becoming perceptive in his elder years. "I also notice you and Jacquie reach across the recliners to touch or hold each others hands or arms Don." He's getting fresh but he is correct. I heard an elder counselor state that the elderly do not get enough touching. At least we're working on it.

I notice other seniors have scaled back on the type of fireworks they use. The lucky ones have found new interests. Keeping busy and interested in others or in an avocation is a key to senior happiness, it appears.

One misfire occurred this Monday evening, at bed-making time. When I was a kid on the farm, we worked until it was too dark to see in the field before coming home to the farmstead. Then it was a drive to the pasture, often rounding up the cows by car light before milking, and then home again to separate the milk. By the time the hogs were fed, Mother had supper ready. It was time for bed, but the beds weren't made. Mother had been attending a meeting, working in her large garden or canning food. I was tired, and swore if I was ever in charge of bed making, I would do it as soon as I got up. Now that JJL is ill, I make the bed whenever she leaves it. There was an exception Monday.

As she arose JJL said, "Don't make the bed Don, I want to change it." She was feeling better and while I am rather good at making the bed with Mocha's assistance, I decided JJL would feel better about herself if she helped to make it. She is beginning to feel bad about having to depend on me so much. You guessed it! She didn't get ready to make it until after the eleven o'clock news. I was quite tired as I went to the bedroom and remembered the boyhood promise I made to myself.

"Here are the clean sheets," my wife said throwing them onto the bed. I don't know if Mocha understood not, but she landed on the bed almost simultaneously with the sheets. She did understand what was to happen next, I'm sure, as she began to do rolls and jumps around the still unstripped bed. I rolled her over a time or so, and her frenzy increased. She was covered by the first clean sheet but only for a moment. After a roll or two she positioned herself to help with the top sheet. The whole process was repeated again with the comforter. "It's been fun," she meowed with her soft voice as she looked up at me.

I crawled into bed after undressing and getting JJL ready for bed. Mocha came to me and lay in the space below my arm. I petted her. She turned and backed into my armpit with more soft comments. She does not have hair fastened to her flesh like most cats. Hers is a loose pelt, and she likes me to manipulate it with vigorous movements of my fingers. Most people know that scratching a puppy in the right place under its chin will cause it to do a series of kicking. I wasn't thinking about that as I moved my finger massage up and down Mocha's back, and then it happened! I hit a spot I had not known about. It caused her to empty her bladder in one spontaneous shot! This five-inch zone of warmth came through the comforter and the sheet, onto me, and of course onto the bottom sheet. It was time to remake the bed, even before Jacquie was in it. Mocha did not help us this time. She was fifteen feet away doing her own wash-up.

Hereafter I will stroke her coat lightly when she settles on the bed beside me.

I didn't know it then but I would soon hear my name called in a plea for help and we would be seeing our nice little doctor Banda again. I had my appendix removed decades ago but I now try to convince the doctor I have grown another and it is causing my bellyache.

Chapter 19

Am I Going Down for the Count?
Aging Can Mean Mature Confusion

Will I get used to having my name being called in a panicky voice? Self read my thoughts and whispers, "Probably not." Having a spouse who has balance problems and is prone to wandering off without help is not unlike having a toddler exploring its new world.

I remember last evening. Jacquie wandered off and came back from the kitchen cabinet with a bottle of little pills she couldn't open, another childproof, senior-proof device. She brought it to me as I sat in the recliner. I opened the bottle and as I tried to extract a second pill, it jumped and disappeared. We couldn't find it and I got the flashlight. She went behind the recliner and tipped it back while I shined the light under it. And then again those words were said in a frightening manner, "Don, Don!" I looked up and she has fallen between the backs of the recliners. I quickly rose, ran around the furniture and helped her to her feet. It was then Latte surprised us. She is instantly on a recliner back and with a wide mouth puts her teeth upon JJL's arm. She doesn't break the skin, but Jacquie's cry has informed her all is not well and she wants the problem stopped. We have noticed this reaction before. Latte turned her attention to me. I received two wet licks of her tongue before she nipped my arm. Now that she had warned us, she hopped down and went elsewhere.

After turning off the living room TV, our ritual is to go to the kitchen and our mini-pharmacy. Jacquie hands me a sundae glass to receive her pills. She has a re-occurring habit of dropping pills onto our multicolored floor covering. Since she has been ordered to not bend over, it is easy to guess who is labeled as the official pill retriever. She hands me a glass for water, but I take cuts and take my pills first. This may appear to be rude but I have found I forget to take my pills otherwise. My me-first rule solves this problem.

With the pilling complete it was time to move to the next stage of medication, her regular evening insulin shot. I removed the container from the refrigerator and rolled it between my hands to mix the ingredients before cleaning its top with an alcohol pad. I removed the syringe cap to load the needle before handing it to her. We are done, I thought, and I took off my glasses.

"Don, help!" When an aged lady prone to falling talks that way one tends to quickly investigate the reason. "I've dropped my diabetes blood-sugar testing strip and can't see it. Can you help?" I dropped to my knees again after reattaching my glasses. I breathed a prayer of thanks that I have an over-the-counter medication that grows cartilage back into my aching knees. I started looking on the multi-colored floor for the tiny strip.

"I can't find it. I'll get the flashlight." Fortunately the light was nearby and I was soon on the floor again. Mocha arrives to investigate. "Mocha heard us," I announced, as she walked between JJL's legs and into my beam of light.

"She's not going to help you. She just wants attention," my spouse informed me. Yes, she has walked into center stage. We have lights, a prima donna and action.

"Here's your strip. It was never on the floor. It was on your hospital sock." I took off my glasses again and we went to bed.

"Don." There's that attention getting word again. "You need -" an action phrase "to get me another bottle of insulin. How much is left in the one I'm using?"

"It's half full and should last several weeks yet. Besides, you have a second bottle."

"Where?"

"On the shelf with our other spares."

She gets out of bed and I take her to the kitchen to look for it. That bothers me but my word has not been accepted a time or two in out half century of marriage. "Hey, forget it, I'll check tomorrow," I say,

An Old Man

hoping I will remember. This time we do get to bed. Yes, medicating is serious stuff and it occurs every night when I am most tired. Team medicating is a production taking a lot of cooperation, snoopervision, double-checking and some suspicion. It's like Jessica Fletcher, the doctor and the sheriff going over the evidence together.

This morning it doesn't seem that I will get to sleep again after the old man call I answered in the middle of the night. An HMO booklet states that after trying for fifteen minutes to get to sleep, one should choose another activity. I chose to get up, fire up the computer and work on a manuscript about problems Jon and I have found while inspecting new houses. I am having fun writing this history. While the silicon chips are awakening and flexing their microns, I put a cup of instant coffee and water into the microwave.'

Now back to the computer armed with my hot brew. The manuscript I am working on is about what I look for in a house inspection. It includes a number of graphics and drawings. I find it fun and challenging to set margins, install text boxes, work with underlining and other formatting and creating graphics. Even better, the printed copy looks nicer than the monitor version.

An hour later I look out my studio window and note the sky is lightening. It is time to heed the advice my doctor gave me yesterday at my yearly physical: "Don, I want you to keep walking. Walk everyday. I mean it!" So, putting on a light jacket and my old white cloth hat so motorists not quite awake can see me, I start across the crosswalks. It is that interesting time of the day when dawn is just about to enter center stage. Streetlights are not unanimous in deciding when dawn arrives. They don't have a spouse to tell them when they can turn off, so they are on their own. Some are early quitters while others shine on a few minutes longer before going to sleep.

Eighteen contrails are backlighted by the yet-to-be-seen rising sun. It must have been a busy night of flying or the upper air is still. It is six AM and the street is filling with commuters.

I buy a few things we need and carry them in two plastic bags so the load on each arm is the same. Heading home, I see an early workman with just enough light to see the nails he is pulling out of curbing forms. He is starting very early.

Crows have left their roosts and are standing on the tops of light standards all down the street. It must be too early for pigeons as none are in sight. Maybe like the lady I will see at a Realtor marketing meeting in an hour, they needed a wake-up call. This lady was oversleeping so her husband in the kitchen fixing breakfast pulled out his cell phone and called her on her upstairs bedside instrument.

Now I head home to fill the two weekly pillboxes. With the millions of Baby Boomers becoming seniors pharmaceutical stocks look to be good buys.

Two days later the dawn fools me. It is Monday and it looks like the week is starting in a top-of-the-line fashion. It doesn't continue that way. It is the first of several bad days for me and in fright I wonder if I am going to become an old man. Could I be history at just seventy-five?

JJL is not beyond doing some supervising so we are doing some little pick-up chores around the house. "Pick up <u>your</u> cat's hair on the recliner. <u>Take</u> the water glasses from last night to the sink." She excels at delegating and I'll give her an A grade in that. "<u>Did you</u> bring in the Sunday paper?"

"It's Monday," I correct her, at least in theory.

My dad used to say, "If convinced against your will, you're of the same opinion still."

"She is having more memory problems," Self says, underlining the thoughts I'm having.

I say something about an experience she had in the hospital and she doesn't remember it. So I get out my writings for class and read her my humored version of the various escapades and events she had there. Most of it is news to her. As I read about a throat specialist massaging her throat and the language he used in an attempt to increase the opening size, she remembers. Her description is, "Excruciation and a never-to-do-again thing!" Her memory is on track about that episode.

It is time for the 49ers' football game and I am glad to sit down. The Oakland A's are in a play-off game at one so I can continue to sit. I'm not feeling my best. In the evening, we'll watch the Oakland Raiders. After two large spoonfuls of potato salad I made yesterday and some rice pudding, I persist in my do-nothing mode. I am glad to sit still for a change. "I'll charge my batteries and really go tomorrow," I tell myself. How wrong I am.

At halftime, in the Raiders' game, I notice my right groin is hurting. By the end of the game I'm miserable, about seven or eight on the ten-point pain scale of my HMO. "I'll take an aspirin and go to bed if you can take your bedtime medicine and inject your insulin," I tell JJL. What I don't tell her is that I'll take three aspirins, chew them and wash the grains down with a glass of water. I am almost desperate, but am soon asleep.

At two-thirty the pain cuts through the sleep and awakens me. The aspirins have worn off. I lie awake until three, then get up and dress in my only long-sleeved shirt. I put on a coat before sitting in the recliner, and cover my lower parts with a blanket. I am cold and miserable. At three-thirty I get the HMO customer's bible about health and read about possible causes of abdomen pain. It states I could be constipated, dehydrated or pregnant. My appendix left me a half-century ago and I am taking my stress medicine. It also says time isn't too important, but to call if the pain continues. At five-thirty I phone the advice nurse and go through the reasons for pain with her. She doesn't panic, but tells me to call for a doctor appointment after the appointment center opens at six-fifteen. She says I can take a pain prescription I've had awhile after I check its expiration date. At six-thirty I set up my appointment and one for JJL, whose last fall is still bothering her neck.

At the doctor's clinic, we each have an x-ray and I have two blood draws after I lose my argument with the Doctor Banda. I tell her I have grown a new appendix and it is infected. The look in her pretty dark eyes tells me in no uncertain terms that I'm not even in the right playing field.

Walking hurts me. Our trips around the facility are a problem to me even before JJL starts having a new problem herself. "My walker wants to go to the right. I can't control it," she says, handing it to me to carry along with her purse. She needs both hands to hold onto me as we go for her x-ray.

"You need a two-seated wheelchair Don," Self chides.

Arriving home at seven that evening, I take one of the pills for my now diagnosed case of diverticulitis and head for bed while JJL heads for the TV. I am hurting, tired and soon asleep. It seems only minutes later that I hear noises in our bedroom and a scraping noise in the kitchen. That would be her walker on the floor, I think. Cracking an eye, I check to see what is going on in the darkened bedroom. Before I see anything there is a crashing noise at our folding closet doors.

With both eyes now open I see my spouse headed across the end of the bed in a jerky manner. "Having trouble?" I ask.

"Yes. I've fallen many times but not to the floor. I almost fell with the walker and I nearly ended up in the sunken tub. I fell against the closet doors." She had trouble walking to her x-ray earlier. Did she miss her travel medication for dizziness or is she having another mini-stroke?

"I'll get up and help you."

"No, you're sick. I'll get your second antibiotic and be back." I feel confused; not sure whether I should fight her concern for me, I let her go. "Is this the one?" she soon asks. Sitting up and reaching for my glasses, I am glad to say it is the right medicine before taking it and the water she has somehow carried with the walker. I take off my glasses and lean back into bed again.

Turning she says, "Now I need to get my new medicine." She is gone but only for a minute. She appears at bedside with another bottle of medicine. "Is this mine?" I get my glasses again. "It is, Jacquie."

She has another concern. "Don, we need to put the drops in my ears so the wax can be taken out when we go to the nurse tomorrow. Where is the bottle? I can't find it." I am still hurting rather badly and do not enjoy getting up to look for the bottle. I get up and don't find it so back to the bed stand for my glasses. I find the hiding bottle in plain sight in the middle of the dining table. I think all will be well as I hand the wax softener back to my nurse for the evening.

All is not well with her. "I can't get the little pull-off cap to pull off." It is yet another of those childproof, senior-proof containers. After helping her, I lay back to go to sleep without glasses. It seems only a moment later when she again appears. "Please remove the ends of my insulin syringe. I've tried four of them and can't get any to come off." More childproof containers! I would guess this medicine routine is repeated in many homes and is a part of life's October. We will get to sleep. We will. And we do.

I have a bad dream. It is about a broken tractor I own. I take it to Kansas for repairs. The universal joint is re-welded and I come back to California. After awakening this morning I read the cautions on my new medicine. "It may cause interesting dreams!"

I have another medical problem a night later. My wife is in bed and I need drops in my ear. While I can't count five drops, as I can't

An Old Man

see my ear, I can feel the coldness as they entered it. Oops, I've used too much. I look at the bottle and absentmindedly, instead of pulling off the tip; I've unscrewed the cap and poured the liquid in the ear. I awaken in the night to notice a spot on the sheet and then I see another spot. Is it blood from my ear? It takes a little more awaking to realize we are sleeping on a patterned sheet. This is not a dream!

The upshot of these episodes is that for a day or so neither of us has a decent caregiver. I guess we are fortunate to have only a short time of it. And the younger generation believes growing older means only walking more slowly and not as far.

The funny thing is how we generalize about everything. One of JJL's hospital roommates passed a driving test at eighty-nine and Dr. Grace is driving at ninety-six. I've never followed either of these ladies, but they must do better than a much younger senior we saw last week in a shopping center. I was in the center lane when I saw this lady approaching on the right. I slowed and watched her drive over a stop sign painted on the pavement and cut in front of me. Two hundred feet later she drives over another stop sign and passes in front of a lady turning across her. That lady too, is observant and gives way. I notice the errant driver's nearly new car has no dents or scratches. She must own a good body shop!

My medicine corrected my problem and I'm up the next day and at the computer. I've composed, typed, backspaced, and now I'm tired. While the antibiotics are working slowly or perhaps older bodies respond slower, I'm tiring. It's still dark so I'll lie down before redressing to take my puzzles to the local Realtor meeting. In other words, I'll conserve my strength.

It is warm for the month and later we'll have a senior matrimonial disagreement. As I was going to turn on the AC, JJL asks, "Turn on the furnace please." This getting older is something else! Some scientists want to enable us to live longer. Sometimes I wonder why. I can't rollerblade, stay awake in the evenings or stay asleep all night.

Will things get better or continue to disintegrate? Somethin's goin'ta hafta change!

Chapter 20

The Blue Moon Halloween
The Quiet Before It Comes Apart

It is a blue moon I'll always remember. I just have learned blue moons are the second full moon of a month. This one in October is special. It occurs on Halloween, an event that won't happen again until 2020. But most important, it is maybe the most important happening in my life recently. Like ending the October month on the calendar this night might be ending my life's October. Upon awakening I find my life becoming November-like. It is the time of fall to set the clock back an hour to regular time. I am glad. It gives me another hour of lifetime or am I grasping for straws. If my death call comes on Daylight Savings Time, that will shorten my life by an hour.

Why do I wonder about November? I'm not a prophet. If I were a prophet, I wouldn't wonder, I would know. On Halloween I find myself sidestepping twice to maintain my balance. This happened also yesterday, two days in a row. I'm a septuagenarian, and walking difficulties are to be expected at this age; however, I walk three miles a day and when I had a physical two weeks ago, I was found to be in good health.

One expects to replace a transmission or a radiator in an old car. Will I need a new balance or guidance chip before long? My attitude is good and I try to walk as if I am only fifty-five, head up and a with a purposeful stride. My doubts start when for three days in a row I find I have little motivation to start or continue the day, an unusual condition for me. Do I need a new starter also? My wife Jacquie's main complaint is that I can't sit still. I always have to be doing something. I'm a wiggler and a doer. Well, those three days of feeling uncharged and sitting beside her may cause happiness for her, but they are downers for me. Am I entering November and shifting into a lower gear? I hope not. I plan to run right up to my grave, or at least jog. Is this tiring of mind and body a natural function of aging? Do I need to take bigger vitamins or take them more often?

While I usually waken between four and six to get up for writing, I awaken now without any strength, not caring about turning on the word processor. Something is terribly wrong. Is the internal computer that governs my days malfunctioning? I wonder if I need one of Jacquie's pills to make me sleep longer. I have some sleeping pills, but I want to know more about them. How long will they cause me to sleep? Can I be awakened easily? JJL is ill, and I need to hear any calls for help. She falls too often, and I want to accompany her about the house, even though she uses a walker. Her last fall was the worst yet. She has exceeded any quota for falling and appears to be going for a new record. Is this worry tiring me? Does my tiredness result from stress?

"I'll bet it does," Self whispers. "You need to remember you're a caregiver. Don't let yourself get down."

His flippant remark causes me to do some reflecting. It's been quite a bad summer for her. In fact, she left the October of her life and entered November several months ago, rather abruptly, when she had those mini-strokes, her series of emergency room visits and hospital stays. She now needs care, and I'm her only caregiver. I function as washerman, cook, nurse, assistant in dressing and undressing, medicator and the like. I am also the necessary scapegoat when things go wrong. I manage yard care, housekeeping and the marketing of the family business as best as I can. Fortunately, I am healthy, but as any caretaker will attest, the process can be wearing. The Internet has many articles validating the fact. Care giving is an underrated malady.

After learning of JJL's condition, many people talk to me about the stress of care giving. They shake a finger at me and tell me to take care of myself. "You'll not do her any good if you let yourself get down," they warn. The looks in their eyes emphasize it. "I mean it, Don," a Realtor with care giving experience tells me this morning. For once in my life I will heed female advice given me.

Self, who hasn't said much for awhile, now opens up on me once again. "I think too much stress is your problem. It just might be manifesting itself differently then it did than the night of your ambulance trip. Can stress express itself as lethargy as well as pain?' If I have time, I may look up a health web site or e-mail the doctor who is a part of the six o'clock TV news team and check that thought. Self may be right.

Now, in addition to watching my blood pressure, my caloric intake and my miles of walking, I need to watch my stress level and plan accordingly. I wish there were a machine for that. If I live long enough, it might be a challenge for me to develop one. Not even the doctors have such a device.

"Think of the market!" Self says aloud.

As I walk in the dawning light today, I think of a new game I could develop for people with stress. Cards would name different kinds of stress and have values accordingly. The commute cards could vary from the glaring orange card of "Three Right Lanes Blocked" to a yellow card, "Running Low on Gas," or a gray one, "Medium Visibility." Other cards about life at home could be "No TP in the Bathroom," "What's for Dinner?" and "The Pantry's Empty." A version for seniors would have cards like "Out of Pills," "Where'd I leave my Cane?" "What day is it?" "Where are my hearing aides?" and " I have only one shoe on."

The dawn walk seems to help my stress level. As I set out, the eastern sky is beginning to lighten. Then the Morning Star peeks over the hills to the east with its low wattage half-brother baby star in tow. I wondered if this is called a, "star rise?" The sea gulls are heading west so we'll have a nice day, according to an old sailor's saying. The fresh air feels good and acts as a relaxing stress medication. "Fall is a great season," I tell my wife each year. "It must be female. It is beautiful, colorful, fickle and changeable." My partner of few words wrinkles her nose and sticks out her tongue at me

I get a more vocal response when I tease workers stocking shelves at Safeway. I answered one's, "Have a good day, Don," with, "Don't do anything I wouldn't do and you'll be OK."

She retorted, "I'll do anything you'd do and I'll do it better!" She must be someone's wife. Hats off to her! She relaxes me a bit. I chuckle about her reply several times on the walk home. Chuckling is a good relaxing medication and best of all it's over-the-counter and easy to take.

With plastic shopping bags containing Jell-O, cottage cheese, rice, and a package of hamburger, I stride from the store and up the railroad overpass. I look to see how high my two stars have climbed while I shopped. I am disappointed; they have gone to bed. The dawn has brightened. Stars have been upstaged by the light from the soon-to-be-seen sun. This footlight effect is warming the valley's silhouette of dark hills into a softening stage setting for what appears to be a nice day. The dawn is becoming noisy as well as light. There is the roar of a nearby freeway, and the whoosh of traffic on the streets leading to it.

Then another voice enters the din. The Altamont express train is quietly coasting down the pass and into town. I see commuters with their laptop computers, cell phones and briefcases in the well-lit cars. As the train disappears under me I turn to descend the over-crossing and I notice my knee does not hurt as it has for the past month. The over-the-counter pills are helping me grow more cartilage. That slowing down I noted days ago must have been the result of a bug of some sort, as this morning I feel almost back to par. "It will be a good day, Self. Help me be positive."

"I'll do what I can, Boss."

A walk can provide an opportunity for a lot of uninterrupted thought. We septuagenarians have a lot of memories that can be dusted off easily and re-enjoyed. It is fun living in the past: few risks are taken, little energy is required and we don't need an audience or any gadgets. This morning finds me asking myself futuristic questions: Where's JJL's health going? Is she really getting a bit better? Or are my subconscious wishes affecting my observations? Perhaps she is on a plateau. Am I doing as well as I can for the both of us? Thank goodness they were mini-strokes rather than maxi-strokes, I tell myself, with a heavenward look, as I add, "Thank you." The scripts for seniors to play can be quite varied and can change even as one walks onto center stage. My Jacquie will have to walk farther into our script before we know her role in the future. She continues to mystify the medics and me.

Turning off Colgate Way onto Lincoln Avenue I have one last thought as I spot our house. JJL is a little better than she was four months ago when her health changed and no one seemed able to help us. I should check some of the health sites on the Internet for mini-strokes to see what more I can learn. Since I need to be at the house much of the time, the Internet will work fine. I will find more information than I could at the library.

Maybe I should add care taking, stress and aging to my Web search list as well. If I find anything I want to remember, I will print it with my computer, since the bypass operation did affect my memory, a common side effect, as I was warned the night before the operation..

In a newly developed procedure the chest is not opened which eliminates that brain damage risk. Three openings are made. After inert gas expands the chest to give room, a light and camera on a tube are inserted through one opening. Two other openings allow rods holding scalpels and needles to do the surgery. The doctor watches what he is doing on a color monitor on the wall: a modern miracle! The recovery time is much quicker, I hear, and the brain doesn't suffer.

On my entry walk to my front door, I pick up our paper and am greeted with, "Hi there. Good morning." It is Jake and her walking partner, a half block away. I don't know these ladies, who are in their mid-thirties, but we have been exchanging street greetings for several months when we meet in the early dawn walks. They are too busy to visit with me today, so a short conversation ensues as they stride purposefully past me and on up the hill.

I am lucky to have incidental friends. I regularly converse with the Safeway produce man who fluffs his bin of string beans to give them a better presentation to shoppers. The meat man filling his display case and a young checker also pass the time of day with me and we exchange smiles, a great way to start the day. In an hour I will be enjoying chitchat with Realtors and their affiliates in another county. More smiles.

Years ago we were wise to buy an insurance policy for long term care. A lady has been funded to come several days a week to help me with JJL. This lady is Jane who has been doing our laundry and house cleaning for a year. Like JJL she doesn't do much talking so they get along fine. While JJL sleeps or watches TV, Jane sits nearby, ready to help her to the bathroom or get a glass of water.

Having Jane for two four-hour sessions a week lessens the stress I feel. I can step out of my strict regime now and then. I schedule my trips to market the family company business on the days the caretaker is with Jacquie. This allows me a chance to get away and meet friends and colleagues. Perhaps all is set for me but if I am stumbling into my

November, I need to be alert to stay on top of what is ahead. "It's good I have Jane, the caretaker," I tell Self with a slight smile. "And our cats, Latte and Mocha are like family. I'm not bad off."

"Those felines have played an important part in your JJL's bounding back a bit from her worst time. Don, I also think they help you keep your stress in check."

"I need to take more time to play with them for both their and my sakes. Time petting and listening to their purring will help us all."

I look for and do find joy in my everyday life. Mocha, my Birman feline, talked with me as we had our quality time earlier, but she is quiet now as she lies beside me on her towel. "I am blessed," I tell her as I stroke her one more time before transferring my hand from cat to computer mouse. Legend has it that the soul of a dying monk of one sect is reborn as a Birman cat. Perhaps that is why my relationship with Mocha seems more than an animal to human relationship. She is a close and caring individual.

Outside my studio window a brazen scrub jay with a fast glide arrives on the patio where I have scattered feed for the ground-feeding birds. Without hesitation, he seems to say, "Don put out some shelled peanuts this morning. Good for him and me too." He checks each pile of seed for the peanuts, which he'll carry to someone's yard to bury. Sparrows arrive, but they observe pecking protocol and stay away from the jay's self-imposed territory. Mr. Jay takes three quick bounces and flies away, allowing the sparrows to approach the serve-yourself breakfast table. As feeding starts, a dove without tail-feathers comes near, approaches, but is intimidated by a rapidly feeding sparrow family. It is good they eat fast, as two jays swoop into the yard with landing gear down and body language shouting, "We'll take over here!"

I return my attention to the keyboard. I need to write several paragraphs about an interesting Christmas gift I have given or received. This is my assignment for the writing class Christmas party tonight. I thought about this last night as I went to sleep, so my planning is done. Watching the jay in the back yard reminds me of an interesting gift that fits the assignment.

As I start to write, Mocha joins me. While she has learned to avoid stepping on the keyboard, she sometimes missteps and my screen changes rather interestingly. It is not hard to forgive her, as she is purring, and she rubs against me as she lifts her foot from the key she offends. The most disturbing aspect of her affection is her fluffy tail rubbing across my nose, which makes me sneeze. Now to the short sharing tidbit for the party tonight.

A Nutty Christmas

I was nine years old and we were just coming out of the great depression on the plains of Kansas. While the Chinese designate years of the dragon or the pig, we Jayhawkers designated Nineteen Thirty Six as the Year of the Grasshopper. The crop-devouring plague of insects was compounded by a drought. I was old enough to realize this Christmas would not yield a great harvest of gifts. Mother and Dad had both had their teeth pulled, and went for a year before they could afford false replacements. Visa and Master Card were not available and conservative mid westerners were a cash-and-carry breed: no cash, no carry!

Christmas toys were conservative in both size and number in those days. As times were hard, there had not been much money for treats, either. After the country school Christmas program, we knew we would get a sack of candy, containing a nice orange, several sugarplums, some striped pieces of ribbon candy, silver pillows filled with black walnut, and perhaps some nuts, courtesy of the school board. If you were in the church program Christmas Eve, you would receive another paper sack with the similar treats.

On Christmas morning that year I found a large brown grocery sack under our tree with my name on it. It must be a hard-to-wrap toy, I thought. It was squeezable and had no weight. Maybe there was excelsior around a breakable toy. I pulled off the top covering and found the sack to be filled with peanuts in the shell. I was very pleased, as my folks reacted to my surprise with large smiles.

After school I would park my tin dinner pail, fill my Mackinaw coat pockets with peanuts and go outside to do the chores. It was great. You could drop peanut shells in the farmyard, the barn or in a corral and not be scolded. What a nutty and memorable Christmas!

As I spell-check this short subject, I hear the tinkling of a bell. JJL is awake and needs my help. I hit the print icon and head for the bedroom. She probably needs some water and pain pills. With her eyes still shut, she raises an arm above her head and extends two fingers. I go to the acetaminophen bottle for two capsules and check that her bedside glass has water. She will go back to sleep, and I will need to fill medication boxes for daily dosages for the week ahead. More work on the computer will probably have to wait.

The medication "roulette ritual," the counting of many medications into the proper sections of the week's dispenser compartments for each of us takes about an hour per week. Some pills have to be cut, while others are dispensed as several pills per dose. Perhaps I should set up a business of picking up medicines from the pharmacy, counting them into proper daily doses and sealing the containers before delivering them to elderly patients. It's done that way for nursing home patients. With all the baby boomers reaching the years when the number and frequency of medication increases there's a lot of counting in the future.

Chapter 21

Sitting? No!
Sitting With A Reason
Am I Changing?

It's morning again. I've lived in two centuries, in nine different decades, but I'm thinking I've never enjoyed mornings more than now. After all this time I've learned to increase my appreciation of what mornings have to offer. I've always enjoyed the physical happenings, the coloring of the sky, the sound of birds, the wind and the smell of the cool air. After awakening before dawn, I take my cup of coffee to that old red rocker and let my senses and imagination run as they choose.

This morning I realize the sounds around me in the darkened house are quite interesting. The comfortable thump of the furnace beginning its workday reaches me from across the house. I like that sensation. I am halfway through the coffee when Mocha arrives, greeting with a soft "Merrr." She rubs against me, offering her second communication for my senses to enjoy, but she is not finished. She hops down, and a moment later I hear a noise and sense a dark object behind her as she dashes past the Christmas tree we've put up days before Thanksgiving. There is just enough light to see that she is dragging an old shaggy pillow to the middle of the room. She makes a thump as she tries to dive under the pillow. As I turn in the chair, there is a small rustling beside me. My sock foot has bumped against the wrapping of a present under the tree. I am enjoying the sounds in the darkness of this morning.

Yesterday I turned on the Christmas tree lights and sat beside it in the dark, feeling silent joy and satisfaction. With a pair of cats, one can have an interesting visual experience each morning before Christmas, looking to see which tree ornaments have to be re-hung. Putting up the tree was a challenge. I was having several days of tiredness, and JJL couldn't help with the tree erection, so we called our grandson, Drew to help us. Drew is Jon and Donna's son. After the tree was assembled, I was tired, so we postponed the decorating for a day. It also meant we would see Drew for two days. Then, with more strength, I provided a chair for JJL. Sitting in it she unpacked the decorations and told Drew which ones needed to be above the reach of the cats. Drew is tall enough that a stepstool was not needed to place the top ornaments. It was a cooperative effort and enjoyable. JJL felt more of a sense of accomplishment than she had for some time. Yesterday I sat more than usual, and enjoyed the sensation of another dawn. The increasing light of the sun painted the undersides of the clouds with the colors of a warm pallet. Yes, I am enjoying my mornings more than in the past.

Screen and video writers colossalize everything, and we have been conditioned to expect a lot of spectacular things in life. "If it's not spectacular, it's not worth much," seems to be their message. I find myself conditioning my senses to enjoy greatly the little happenings in life. For example, at a holiday party I watched the ladies organize the food on the serving table as they perceived how it should be arranged. One self-appointed helper re-cut the pie after the lady who brought the pie divided it. Parties are a great place for the noble sport of people watching. I drove home with a smile on my face, not about spectacular happenings, but remembering interesting details of a pretty simple party.

Jacquie also gives me some laughs now and then but sometimes the situation rubs me the wrong way. An example is when Latte is asleep on her lap, either on the bed or recliner. My wife will say, "I wish she would wake up."

"Do you need to go to the bathroom?"

"Yes." A cat needs eighteen hours of sleep a day, but it is permissible to awaken them when the adult has a need also.

"I'll move her to the pillow on the chair over there."

Then I find I need instructions to move the cat for the tenth time this week. "Don't hurt her! Be careful and don't hurt her," as if I would.

I find the intimation that I might hurt Latte interesting at times and irritating at other times. Then I remember her actions can be the result of TIAs, often called, mini-strokes. If only we had seen the signs, Jacquie might be in better shape.

There will be other signs and only days away. Her next misfortune will ruin the Thanksgiving dinner plans I was preparing for the family.

Chapter 22

She Does It Again But Head First This Time!

"Oh, No, Jacquie!"

It is a beautiful morning this Tuesday before Thanksgiving, in fact, too nice a morning for a fall, especially a bad one.

JJL has headaches that last most of each day. Fortunately, several months ago the headache clinic was able to stop the worst ones, migraines that had affected her every day for several months. I found the clinic two towns away, listed on the Internet. It is affiliated with our HMO but in another jurisdiction, so Doctor Banda didn't know of it.

JJL spends her days in the recliner except for a few times when she feels like walking with me for three or four blocks. Her balance problem requires that she holds my arm, and we walk slowly. On this morning she reminds me, "The forecast is for rain. Don't you think you had better rake leaves so the drain on the patio doesn't clog and flood?" The TIAs affected the balance portion of her brain but not the administrative and supervisorial segments.

"OK," I say. She should get some outside air, I reason in spite of the Stay Out of the Sun labels on several of her medications, so I add, "Hey, Jacquie, let's get you fresh air while I rake. There is shade under the long overhang of the bedroom so you won't be in the sun." After helping her up and into her walker, I take her through the sliding door, saying, "I'll get you a chair,"

"No, I want to stand," she replies in a very direct tone of voice, and moves several feet to a nearby fuchsia bush. A hummingbird thinks she is too close to his liquid pantry and he buzzes her. She takes a step up onto the next level of the brick patio to look around. I glance at her from the corner of my eye from time to time, and all appears fine.

After a while, I sense she is shifting her walker. A fraction of a second later I realize she has lost it and is falling sidewise over the left side of her support. She goes headfirst over the small planter step. Twisting as I rise to my feet, I'm not able to reach her in time to help. I hear a sickening thump as her forehead hits the bricks of the lower level. She must have passed out prior to falling, and being relaxed may have helped her with the landing. She made no attempt to reach out with her hands to break her fall. That probably prevented broken bones.

She is face down. When I roll her onto to her side she revives and says she is dizzy. Blood is running from her right temple toward her right ear, and as I wipe it away, I see deep abrasions on her temple and a bit of torn flesh on her cheekbone. How did this happen when she was falling to her left?

After a quick wash-up, we go to the small emergency room at the HMO for evaluation. We're told she is not as bad as she looks. Butterfly bandages are affixed to hold the torn cheek flesh in place.

I tell the doctor that the three-times-a-day travel sickness pills prescribed two months ago by someone else had reduced but not stopped her dizziness. This doctor said, "Cut the dosage to once a day, as the stuff can become addictive."

"You know, doctor," I say, "you should order a new A drive to insert in her head, one with a flaw free vertigo program."

He says, "I wish I could."

"Why not? You install new hip and knee joints."

We go home again, with stronger painkillers for this new source of headaches. JJL has half of her forehead and one cheek damaged and crisscrossed with butterfly bandages, and we know the bruise coloring will present a Halloween mask-like appearance not only for Thanksgiving but for many days to come.

I cancel our family dinner I had planned. I had invited Jon, Donna and Drew together with Karen and Darrel. Their son, Eric, his wife, Michelle, and son, Brian were to come also. Jacquie didn't want anyone to see her bandaged and swollen face so we didn't go to the dinner Karen substituted at her ranch. We are a social contrast. I go out of my way to visit with others and my Jacquie has grown quite timid over the years. She will dread a family gathering but enjoy it once she is there.

I suggest eating out but she thinks it would be nice for us to eat alone with our good china and a nice menu. So, while delivering reports the day before Thanksgiving while Jane is with JJL, I stop at several stores looking for the tinned spiced fruits we enjoyed decades ago. I find none, but I do find a small jar of spiced apples, dyed green. I make a nice condiment tray and fix dressing and gravy to go with our chicken and noodle main dish. There is pumpkin pie and we enjoy ourselves. Our daughter comes by later in the day after her dinner party concludes. Since Karen is a very busy executive and we seldom see her, this hour visit was much enjoyed. Other than enduring a serious case of face-and-neck bruising my wife has a good day.

We are in for a long period of healing. When we were kids, our skins healed quickly, but that is not true in the second childhood. The skin at her hairline begins to turn the yellow and green of a wild canary, the under-chin takes on the colors of a cardinal, while her lower neck turns the colors of a bluebird and a blackbird. Within hours her scuffed-up temple was half covered with dark scabs and the discoloration had spread across the right part of her face, accompanied by dark rings around the eyes suggesting she belonged to the raccoon family

We are glad there are no broken arms or other bones. Getting around in a walker when you are dizzy is bad enough with two good arms. If she had hit the corner brick with her eye, the results could have been quite bad.

The Saturday following the fall, JJL's headaches are still quite severe and the over-the-counter and prescription products do not help much. I call the HMO advice nurse, hoping to turn up a solution that will lessen the aches. The nurse listens and after asking questions, she does have some advice. "Since she didn't have a CT scan or x-rays last Tuesday, I think she should come to the ER for further consultations. Can you get her in the car and bring her?"

"Yes," I answer.

"Do it then, and good luck." I like the ladies assigned to the advice nurse role.

"Well not always," Self reminded me. "Have you forgotten the turkey in nurse clothing or visa-versa?"

"I forgot her."

It is hard to dress and move a person in pain, but we take it slow and are soon in the waiting room. People waiting their turn for help glance at JJL's head and then shift their eyes away, as if saying to themselves, "My problem hurts but I look better than she does!"

When it is JJL's turn to go into the little confessional room, she tells her story and after some questions, she is sent for a CT screening. I accompany her gurney to the lower floor and wait outside the screening room. I ask Self, "Is there a chance of her going back to a different room as happened several months ago?"

He replies, "There is that chance," and it happens. The man transporting the gurney starts to put her into a C room, which holds patients for hospital admission. JJL is sharp enough to catch the mistake and tell him she is to go back to the B section of emergency where he got her originally.

Later, we learn that there is no bleeding or damage inside the skull that would cause problems like headaches. I'm not a doctor, but I wonder about hairline cracks to the thin frontal part of skull. If there are hairline cracks, they could be painful, and there is probably nothing that can be done to lessen the pain other than the pills we already have.

JJL has not been able to do much reading and will have her eyes checked once the healing process seems to be finished. After she complains about her glasses bothering her I check them and find the nose pad hardware needs a slight adjustment when she is able to go for an appointment.

A few days later, while Dr. Banda is reviewing JJL's insulin situation, she brings it to our attention that there is still swelling in the thin flesh over the temple, which could be the cause of the pain.

On the way home, I begin to wonder about Jacquie's threshold of pain. She can smell my cauliflower in the refrigerator, even with the door closed, or an onion on my breath a day after I had eaten a bit of potato salad. I sometimes think she can hear a spider running down the wall in the dark. Could her sense of pain also be sharper than that of other people. I keep the thought to myself and we talk of other things.

After a month the discoloration is gone except for a dime-size scab, and so are the painful headaches. The ones she still has are less intense. We do need to be careful as the vertigo remains especially after she sits or stands up. Whether she walks in her walker or not, I walk beside her and hold her arm. Several months ago the HMO determined she should use a wheelchair and provided us with a new one, which we use outside.

Fortunately, my health and strength is sufficient to meet the demands of assisting her but the stress is telling. I don't have the chest pain like the ones that caused my ambulance ride last summer, but I have a tired shoulder and a back problem every day or so. I have learned to roll-breathe, starting with extending the stomach before the chest and then exhaling through the mouth. I have also learned to stretch and tense before relaxing the legs and arms. My aspirin intake has increased and my sleeping is also affected. My three-mile walks seem to help. Doctors and nurses, as well as people who have been caregivers, have warned me about watching out for myself, as I am no help to her if I go down. And people call these the Golden Years!

It is a relief of both of us that JJL's pain is easing. We believe things are getting better, and that hospital trips will be a thing of the past. The thought of being confronted with hospital food again supports that wish. We will learn we are wrong once again.

Chapter 23

Never Go Barefoot In Your Second Childhood
The Stage is Being Set Again

Hallelujah! I waken and realize I am going to celebrate one more day of life. At my age that's the best thought to start a day. That is one of the benefits that go with aging if you feel at least half-well. I notice my mornings are beginning to differ from those of the past. Lately, I think about my day's agenda before throwing back the covers. A year ago I did this thinking as I got out of bed. I'm certainly slowing down. I used to jump out of bed. Now, I ease my feet over the edge

JJL, son Jon and I built this house thirty years ago, and I think I know where every nail and board is. I walk about in the dark with confidence of no stubbed toes or black eyes. This morning I don't account for Jane, who was here yesterday afternoon. Jane, the part-time caretaker, is a cat-lover also. She arrives at the house and glances around to spot the cats before looking for us. I never have to check to see that cat pans have water or food on the days she works. Now, barefoot in the darkness, I kick a full water pan. "I would have never placed the water pan where I just found it," I tell Self. Water drips from my foot as I walk into the kitchen. Self doesn't reply, but I hear him snickering.

Yesterday morning, again barefooted, I stepped onto a soft ornament the cats carry about the house. I'm glad they didn't knock a wooden soldier off the Christmas tree and drag it into my walkway.

Stepping onto a bit of cold, wet cat food on the kitchen floor in the dark is an alarming surprise. Jane had relocated another pan. She now knows the cats are fed out of my direct walkway to the coffee center, the microwave. One morning I knew JJL had been to the kitchen in the night without awakening me. In the dark, I walked at a brisk pace into her walker. She had forgotten it when she came back to bed. I all but went over the top of it, with a surplus of surprise.

"Why do you walk about in the dark?" Self asks. "You're no longer in complete control around here. You're the only one who doesn't understand that."

"I know my way, and if I turn on lights, I awaken JJL and she asks what I'm doing out there."

I forgot to put my trousers on before going to make my coffee this morning, and immediately I regret it. As I start to spoon some powder into my cup, my leg is attacked by a wet and sandpapery tongue. Without having to look, I know it is Latte between my spread ankles, demanding cuts in line for her breakfast. Before I can set the cup and the jar of instant onto the counter, she loses patience and gives me a soft bite on my bare leg. I do a barefoot two-step and assure her with a downward look that she is next. Like her mistress, JJL, she communicates silently. In a short paragraph, her eyes say, "I'll believe that when I see it!" She would have made some tom quite a wife. I step to the refrigerator taking my ankles out of range, and she sits down to wrap her tail around her feet at her feeding zone several feet away. She smells the food I place before her and then walks away, satisfied that she has controlled me one more time. "Females!" I mutter to Self, who is smirking at the little drama. "Will I ever understand them?" If she had a tom and walked away from a mouse he brought her, there would be a catfight, I'll bet!

Now where was I before being pre-empted, I ask myself. I put extra Folgers into my cup, drown it with water and tell the microwave, "Take over."

Yesterday I enjoyed the hot hydrated crystals in the dark, but today I flip the switch that turns on the Christmas tree lights. I ask Self, "Are lighted trees just as pretty in the dark of morning as they are at night?"

"They are!"

I have several strings of lights; each programmed to flash on different routines. These random patterns are a great accompaniment to my hot coffee as I relax in the old red rocker. Any residual stress is slipping away. Today is going to be a good day. I even forgive Latte's earlier behavior as she strolls by giving me a sidewise glance. It is Mocha's turn to come for some quality time, petting and purring.

I sip my instant slowly, but realize I'm taking longer to finish it than I did a year ago. I also enjoy the old red rocker longer than I did last winter.

"You are changing, Don, and slowing down," Self reminds me, "But it's OK. Don't worry about it."

Is that because I can't go as fast and hard, I ask myself or is it because I am learning to enjoy the little things I used to overlook? My time is running out, so, do I slow down and enjoy what's left, or continue to hurry to crowd in as much as I can?

The cup is empty; the cats have finished their morning romps. They are engaged in their first naps of the day. Latte is back on the bed curled into a sleeping ball of fur between her mistress's legs. She has wiggled to spread those legs to create a wider spot for herself. This caused one of JJL's legs to fall from the bed, so I cover it with a coat so as not to awaken either of them. More care giving! It starts early and doesn't stop.

It is raining now, so I will skip my walk and head for the studio to write several checks. When finished I will then start exercising the word processor keyboard, a favorite morning activity. When Jacquie awakens, we will drizzle and dress her for a doctor appointment, which concerns her diabetes. But it isn't to be. Mocha has arrived on my desk, and wants to show her love by rubbing her head against the top of my pen. I'd like to swat her a good one, but I don't. She's purring and she rubs my hand. Her little mouth appears to be smiling at me. Cats!

"Don!" I respond to my wife by dashing to the bedroom. "I want to go to the bathroom." That means, please carefully move sleeping Latte off her legs. "And don't be gruff with her," I'm told. My day is shifting gears, and it is time to put the word processor to sleep until tomorrow morning. I find it hard to write a consistent story with the many interruptions and the long delays between periods of writing.

There are some interesting moments in our increasing periods of failing memories. As I steer her into the bathroom, Jacquie asks, "Is it Thursday or Friday?"

"Neither. It is Wednesday."

"Prove it!"

I show her the date on the morning paper, and she wrinkles up her nose and sticks her tongue out at me. I'm not much better; I forgot to put on my glasses last week. My eye was itching and JJL said, "Put some of the eye drops doc gave you in your eye." I had forgotten I had them. The eye received two drops, and then began to burn. It burned the rest of the evening. Next morning it was fine. I put on my glasses and squinted at the fine print on the bottle. In time I was able to make out the wording "Use only in the ears!"

I tell Jacquie, "I'm as bad as my Grandpa Winkley." He was always rubbing something from a saucer in the medicine cabinet on his itchy scalp. If you have your glasses off, you don't spill anything on the lenses. He had his off the night it happened. He called, "Mom, oh Mom, what is this?" She had been using some varnish, and for some reason, put what little was left in the medicine cabinet.

"Don, your thoughts aren't high drama. They're getting to be a lot of problems. Why're you spending time on 'em?"

"You're not noticing, Self, that Jacquie and my routines are becoming tighter with less variety. That goes with the Fall months of life. Take Becky and Kriss, Larry's girls in Kansas by Sue, his first wife. These young women have never been around aging grandparents. For all they know life is full of activities: water skiing, football, Halloween, basketball, Christmas, Super Bowl, snow fun and many other eventful activities. Eric and Mel grew up with grand and great grandparents. They know about aging.

"If your activities become more routine, I hope they don't become too boring Don."

"I've always had an active and an inquisitive mind and I'm determined to find interests and challenges right up to the bugle call!"

After putting JJL back in bed and covering her I shift my muscles into relaxation mode in the red rocker. I gaze at my wife returning to sleep and remember the spring and summer months of her life. While staying with Grandpa Winkley my junior year of high school I met this shy little freshman girl. We became acquainted and I found myself gauging my pace to meet her at the corner for the final three block walk to school. In the senior year the infrequent dating began.

When I was a junior at Kansas State she became a freshman there. We married in the summer and I moved this city girl to the farm and had her milking the first week we were there. While I drove to finish my masters in education she ran the tractor and combine and followed Dad as the wheat was harvested.

She was still a shy woman but led the country church choir and later in California played the church organ. We bought a piano and she gave lessons. One of her pupils is a well know concert artist today. Self, who was reading my mind commented, "Do you remember she drove into San Francisco at least once?"

"Yes, but she has not been able to take the stress of being in a city now. Remember how we avoided driving in New York by taking the highway around it? And the same with London."

"It was two or more decades ago she stopped wanting to go to stores or answer the phone or the door. She stopped going to functions with you."

"Oh, I remember. People would ask about her and I gave evasive answers.

Neither of us spoke for awhile and I soon joined JJL and Latte in an early morning nap.

Walking to the kitchen for a drink on awakening, I smile remembering my little barefooted problems earlier. They are funny now. I'm not sure whether the incident to happen next week will seem funny, scary or both.

Chapter 24

Good Morning Or Is It?
Some Mornings Can Be Hectic

My built-in "go-to-the-bathroom" alarm didn't go off as usual at two-thirty, I awakened, anyhow, at half past four. I realize I turned the thermostat down too far on retiring, so I don't get up right away; I just lay back and let my mind wander. The bed feels good so why not enjoy it? With my strict mid western upbringing and background, to enjoy staying in bed is almost a sinful act. Mother wanted Dad out to do chores first thing, even on the snowy winter mornings. He would reply from the magazine he was reading, "Don't you think the cows like to stay in their warm beds?"

"Yes, but someone might come and catch you still in the house," was her reply.

An urge for a hot beverage becomes great enough at the half-hour to move me. Remembering the wet sanding of my ankles the other day, and noticing the chilliness of the room, I slip into old clothes before heading for the kitchen. It is a safe journey without any tree decorations to step on or water pans to kick. I reach for the decaf jar, as I am fully awake and didn't need any caffeine. So far, so good, but it is to change. I punch in 1.50 minutes as always into the microwave's brain and order, "Now." I then go to turn on the Christmas tree lights.

The microwave bell sounds, saying, "It's hot, Don!" It isn't. This unit has it in for me, and plays a game of, "I didn't hear your beverage order clearly, sir."

In my mind I can once again hear JJL tell me, "Don, you should learn to punch in the numbers correctly. It's never failed me." I don't know how I can operate it correctly ninety-five percent of the time and then forget this morning. After doing the same sequence a second time, I have hot coffee, hallelujah!

I remember the good feeling I had yesterday sitting in the dark room looking at the lighted tree. Now, sitting down again, I hear a weird sound. It sounds like a cousin of our new door chime. I open the front door, but no one is there. Wrong guess. One ornament on the tree is a good-sized ball with a horse and sleigh circling a large fir tree. I touch the ornament, and the noise changes pitch. I unplug the ornament, and the sleigh inside the ornament stops, as well as the noise.

Leaning back to enjoy the liquid of my labors, I spot Mocha. I have wondered where she is. It takes a little observation and deduction to figure out the answer. Her face peeks out of the darkness beside Jacquie's chair, and then, very carefully and just as slowly, she extends one forefoot in front of her head. After touching the carpet, she eases over it, and then carefully extends the second forefoot. The movement of her eyes and head signals that she is on high alert status and ready for an instant retreat. It is fascinating to watch her slow motion creeping. The ornament noise frightened her and she is recovering. She always runs under the bed when the doorbell sounds. She circles the tree, checks JJL's shoes beside the recliner and goes back into the darkness of the next room.

As I drain my cup I remember that yesterday had its problems also. I fixed a breakfast of ground turkey in a skillet with a chopped apple, and served it with raisin toast and milk. The first problem was learning that JJL had started to get into her walker, and then she passed out. Luckily she fell onto the bed. When she woke, she wanted me near, so I lay down beside her and before long we were fast asleep. Later after our drizzle, I also had a nap. Maybe I too am entering my November of life. I have more fatigue and do not sleep well. Caretaker stress? I wonder.

Self replies, "Afraid so. Watch it!"

Mocha tries to help my stress by loving me. When I go to my studio, she jumps onto the desk after a noisy take-off from a nearby chair. She rubs my hand with her head, brushes my face with her bushy tail before sitting down in front of me, blocking my view of the monitor. She watches the cursor arrow and tries to reach under the monitor to capture it for me. When the arrow stops, she turns to smile at me. I shake my head, smile back and consider myself lucky. She is relaxing me if I look at her actions properly; otherwise she could be adding to the stress. What a lover!

The second problem is the shower, or drizzle, prior to going to see the doctor. The process does not flow correctly. Grasping each side of Jacquie's nightgown and throwing my arms wide, the snaps part and I have her undressed before she can say, "OOPS." She gathers three towels as we head to the shower. "Why three?" I ask.

"One for the chair so I don't have to sit upon the cold plastic seat." By now she is ahead of me. Pulling the rear slider open, she starts to enter.

"Wait, there's more room if you enter from the front and squeeze between the toilet and the shower," I inform her.

"I can get in here." She steps through the ten-inch space between the glass door and the plastic shower chair. Now I am at a disadvantage to catch her if she falls forward in front of the chair; however, she makes it without falling. Her dizziness has abated. I start the water to the showerhead on the hose and undress. Now in the shower, she asks, "Where's the shampoo?" I don't know and can't see any. Fortunately, I'm not yet wet, and am soon out of the shower. "Look in the top left drawer of the cabinet," she says. Finding my glasses so I can distinguish shampoo from mouthwash, I find it and re-enter the shower to help her. So far, so good.

When dry, she turns to exit as she had entered, through that tiny passage. "Wait, come out the front so I can help you," I plead.

"I got in this way," I am informed and she continues her exit. The shower pan is wet, and I am again at a disadvantage. I reach across the chair to help her step out of the shower pan, and hope to stabilize her once she is on the outside floor. I need to write a new drizzle action plan: (1) I check that shampoo is in place, (2) I undress first and (3) I am in position to guide her into and out of the unit more safely.

I tell her, "Being naked and falling in the shower is the last place you want to be if I have to call 911." She can comprehend that, but grudgingly as she wants to do as she pleases. I don't feel bad continuing, "We must be careful. We're not kids anymore!"

The trip to the doctor goes well for the most part. JJL drags a foot several times on the way to the office. The office staff notes she has a balance problem. There is an insulin correction waiting for her.

The cup of latte we have on the way home sets us up for a nice evening. Even Latte has a bonus that evening. JJL informs me, "She likes fresh water so would you empty her bowl and refill it, please?"

It's another day as I put my empty coffee cup in the kitchen and go to deliver an inspection report to an address in Castro Valley. Tomorrow I'll tell Jon and Donna about this delivery. It went to an address in a new development, and I caused quite a stir delivering it. In fact, the delivery was more exciting than yesterday's drizzle with Jacquie. I found the house, and note that not all the paving was finished in the front. A pot of flowers sat on the step and a car was beside the entry. "The people must be moving in now," I say to Self.

"It looks like it," he agrees.

With the inspection report in hand I pushed the doorbell, with no response. A second push has the same result. Perhaps the owner is on a ladder hanging curtains or installing something, I think. With many new houses we inspect, we open the front door if it is unlocked, and holler, "Anybody home?" I do this now since the door is unlocked. I hear a sound and step in, to be met by a very surprised man.

"Do you always walk into houses?" he says with an odd look on his face.

"No, but I need to deliver this report. Are you the owner?"

"No. The alarm is on and I don't know how to shut it off," he says as he runs to the controls and begins pushing buttons. He is unable to stop the shrieking noise now announcing itself. This fellow appears frightened.

"Maybe I'm interrupting a burglar?" I confide to Self who for once doesn't have a snide remark.

"I've got to see if I can reach the owner," the fellow says as he whips a cell phone from its holster.

As he begins explaining to the lady who owns the house, I hear a woman's loud voice in the next room replace the shrieking. It is very authoritative in manner. I am not frightened, but I wonder what I had gotten myself into. That voice is somewhere high in the ceiling, as if on a ladder, but there is no ladder. The voice asks, "Who's there? What's your name? Why are you there? This is the Security Company. Who are you?"

I realize then why the other fellow is upset, and then I begin wondering who he is. "Don Larsen, and I'm delivering a house inspection report." I probably should have added, "There's someone else here, and he doesn't know the settings for the sensor. Maybe he is a burglar. Send the cops!"

All the noise – the squawking of the security lady, the clanging of the alarm and the shouting of the man into his phone - makes none of the communications very understandable. The second time the lady asks for a name, my fellow occupant shouts at the ceiling, "Harry. I have the owner on the phone and she's telling me how to turn off the alarm." Finally the alarm becomes quiet, as does the security guard. The man also settles down. He tells me he is a relative of the owner and had come in with a subcontractor earlier. He goes back to his paintbrush as I quietly slip out. I should have left the report on the front porch, even though the approaching rain would have hit it. It's hard to play God with a winning hand!

As I push the computer switch this morning, I run over the plans for the day while the chips warm to the computing tasks ahead. Jane will arrive in hours to do the laundry and get the house ready for the weekend. This will be my chance to get away for any errands, as JJL will not be alone. I don't think of any holiday shopping, and anyway, according to the Wal Mart ad on TV last night, the twenty-third of December, "We'll be open till eight on Christmas Eve for any of you last-minute shoppers."

I hear that commercial without any hearing problem, but later I ask, "Huh," once too often

"Get your hearing aids!" JJL shouts. I do, and find her TV is quite loud. I had to turn my aids' volume controls down. I looked and she wasn't wearing her aids. Aging together can be a challenge!

"Having several wives at this stage of life could be quite a challenge, Don," Self informs me after watching this marital exchange. I smile but to myself.

Tomorrow Melanie, our granddaughter, will fly in from Colorado Springs, and she and I can plan Christmas dinner. I know Mel will be a good tonic for Jacquie. As a boy, I noticed Grandma Clara Mae Kannengeiser Winkley would feel much better when relatives came to visit. I'm also looking forward to seeing Mel. She is upbeat and is good medicine for anyone. Mel tonic is easy to take even in big doses.

It is gray outside and chilly. My three females are asleep. Mocha, on her towel beside me, has a paw over her face. She had quite a scare this morning. Her tail quivers several times, she must be dreaming of the complaining noise of the failing Christmas ornament. Latte in bed with JJL, has forced my mate's right leg off the bed, a regular occurrence, it seems. I'm always tucking a bare leg back under the covers or hanging something over the bare leg to keep it warm. I, too, decide to take a nap, as the constant care taking tires me. I will hear JJL when she awakens and calls me, I tell myself. I will hear her. I will. I will!

I don't. Asleep in the recliner, I do not hear her call me. She then uses her walker to make the trip around the end of the bed to the bathroom, and almost has a wreck. She tells me, "I all but lost my balance and nearly went sideways into the sunken bathtub in spite of the walker." That sounds like the fall a month ago. Then she tumbled over the left side of the walker. Today it is the right side. New rule: I need to take naps on the same bed if she is not in the recliner.

She slips out of bed without waking me several days later. Before I am able to post the new rules, I have to call 911. Yes, again.

Chapter 25

An Old Nemesis, 911, Returns Again
An HMO Christmas

It looks as if it will be a great Christmas at our house. As three doctors in the last two months advised that my mate should be placed in a care home, I want to make what might be JJL's last Christmas as a hostess in her own home a great one. Our daughter Karen has offered to host the dinner, but suggests it be at our house with all her mother's good silver, china and crystal. Well, that's the way it's being planned. Really, everything's set. Mel will arrive in time to help me get the turkey started. Karen will arrive soon afterward to lend a hand. I have fun buying a lot of various fruit and vegetables for relish plates, and Donna said she would bring fresh-baked holiday bread. Grandson Eric and his wife Michelle will come, rather than go to her relatives. Jane will be here the afternoon before to tidy the house for the festive event. We don't have a fireplace, so there will be no stockings hung, but otherwise I am ready and JJL concurs, which I find satisfying. All is set. At least, that is the way it's planned for Tuesday, the twenty-fifth. We don't get that far.

Saturday, the twenty-second, Jacquie complains of a pain just below the ribcage. She doesn't want to dress, and I cover her as she sits in the recliner. Sunday is a repeat performance of the malady, and after she has been up for a half-hour, I help her to bed to rest again. No patent medicines or prescriptions for the stomach help. "I will call the advice nurse if the problem continues tomorrow," I promise.

"We'll see!" she says from her bed. It is a long Sunday afternoon, as no football game is played until evening. Since Monday night football would have been on Christmas Eve, it has been moved to Sunday night. The Raiders and 49ers games were moved forward a day and played on Saturday. The day wears on and she is no better.

The same is true Monday morning, I find, after she wakens from the effects of the medication that causes her to sleep till midmorning. "Don't call the nurse!" she says loudly as she sees me pickup the phone. "I don't know what she can do."

It takes time to maneuver through the HMO's maze of automated options. I punched in JJL's patient identification number and finally reach a helpful person. "My wife is in her third day of bellyache," I inform the advice nurse. "What can I do to help her?"

"What medications is she taking?" Answering that is not a problem, as I have our printed list ready whenever I call for advice. "Tell me about the pain. Where is it? How bad is it? Has she ever had a similar pain in the past? Did she eat anything unusual?" This nurse asks a lot of questions; she is apparently reading from a list of bellyache concerns. I do my best to give helpful information, but it is hard to describe someone else's pain. "I can get her in to see her doctor at 1:45 this afternoon. Is that all right?"

I repeat the question to Jacquie, and her vigorous head-shaking and lowered eyebrows indicated it is certainly not all right. "I'm in no mood to see anyone," her eyes proclaim. Some people can read lips, but decades of marriage have taught me to read eyes better.

I relay Jacquie's response. The nurse is silent for a moment. She is not prepared for that answer. She has offered assistance. Then she tells me to...."Hand the phone to your wife." Jacquie is following my part of the discussion, and her head and eyebrow began a repeat performance of objection as my hand with the phone leaves my ear and my eyes take aim at her. "She doesn't want to talk," I inform the nurse. My JJL has avoided the phone for years.

"How can I help if I can't talk to the patient?" the nurse asks, more in a telling tone than a question. Then she commands, "Hand her the phone!" I do and suffer the Jacquie's worst scowl yet. "Mrs. Larsen, are you there?"

"Yes."

"We need to talk if I am to help you. Now," and the questions continued. I am aware of this, as I have picked up an extension. "You need to go to the ER in Walnut Creek. Mr. Larsen, I heard you come onto the line. Can you take her?" I wonder if my wife doesn't like to talk to nurses because, as it is too much like being a husband: questions, answers and orders.

"Yes, I'll get her dressed and bring her."

"By the way," and there are several other inquires. This nurse must have found another list of questions. As she finishes the questions she changes her mind, "No, don't bring her, call 911!"

"I can bring her," I say.

"You can't make the decision. I need to hear the patient make a decision." There must be several blanks at the bottom of her list.

JJL says, "We will come one way or the other," and hangs up. Then, "Don, I need to go to the bathroom, help me." With her seated in the bathroom, I reached for my electric razor to groom my chin.

I notice she is leaning forward while on the toilet her head is moving toward her knees. I put my hand onto her shoulder. It appears she might pitch forward off the fixture. "Are you OK?" I ask. I received only a half grunt. She is slipping out of consciousness. With the other hand, I reach for the bathroom phone and call 911.

Putting the phone down, I hear the front door close. "Jane?" I call.

"Yes."

"Come into the bathroom and help me get Jacquie onto the bed. You pick up her knees and I'll reach around her chest. We'll take her to the bed. I've called 911."

Jacquie is not conscious, and she is challenge to move. Once she is on the bed, I can't get her panty and slacks pulled up, so I ask Jane to adjust them as I put JJL's ankles on my shoulders and lift. "You go ahead with the housework while we're at the hospital."

I let the firemen in the front door, and my sensitive cat, Mocha, seeing these strange-looking firemen, makes a fast scoot under the bed. She had just emerged from running under the bed upon Jane's arrival and it is again back to safety. While one fireman paramedic starts taking blood pressure, blood oxygen readings and pulse on the now-awakening JJL, I give the morning blood sugar level reading and describe the events of the past few minutes to another fellow, who is filling in the situation forms. A neighbor and the ambulance attendants arrive and a gurney is popped into the carrying position.

As the ambulance driver heads for her vehicle door, I ask, "Do you know the way to the highway? When I was taken by ambulance several months ago the driver drove into several courts and a circle before finding a proper route out of our tract."

"Oh yes," she assures me.

I get into our car and head down the hill, although the ambulance driver and the fire truck head up the hill with my wife. I don't see the ambulance at the next intersection or two. The holiday traffic is light, and as I change from one freeway to the other, I tell Self, "Here we go to the hospital again." I begin to sing to myself a song from several decades ago but with different words:

"All I want for Christmas is a con-doe-min, a con-doe-min,

All I want for Christmas is a con-do-min,

Around the corner from a hos-pit-al, around the corner from a hos-pit-al!"

As I finish the tune, I am parking on the third floor of the hospital garage. After a fast walk, I am asking the ER receptionist, "Has Mrs. Larsen been checked in yet?"

"The name isn't familiar. No, she hasn't."

I settle down to wait. In time, she arrives, and I learn that the ambulance driver knew how to reach the freeway to Walnut Creek from the fire station, so she followed the huge, lumbering hook-and-ladder truck slowly back to the station in the opposite direction of the freeway. No wonder I beat her to Walnut Creek!

I started to follow JJL's gurney into the examination room but was told, "Wait until we have her situated." When I could enter and be at her side, I found the ward to be quite crowded. The examining rooms are full, and she is parked beside the nerve center's counter. I brought one of Lillian Jackson Braun's *The Cat Who...* books with me and I began to read it to her while we wait for a room. She has been seen and is receiving an IV, as well as being monitored on an EKG setup. Blood testing is progressing as well. When my eyes need a break from reading I tell her of the condition of some of the folks in the waiting room. There is a medley of wheelchairs and casts. Two young men in leather clothing are splattered with mud. I overhear them tell someone they were having fun in Carnegie Park with their motorcycles climbing the hills after last night's rain. "Boy, it was great!" said the one who is not limping.

In time JJL's name is called. She is seen by a young doctor, who states, "It could be any of a variety of problems, or a combination of several. I'll order some tests."

She is first sent for a CT Scan. I accompany the transporter and his gurney, as it is not only interesting to see other areas, but the hospital misplaced my wife on two earlier stays so I couldn't find her. Surely it couldn't happen again, but I will follow anyhow.

Around a dozen corners, down several halls, past an electric corridor door switch at elbow height, we go to an elevator. Then more halls and a corner bring us to the special room with its shielding and warning signs. In time, the scanning is over and our wheel tracks are retraced, but not back to where we started. The transporter starts to return her to the wrong department. JJL is sharp enough to correct him. That sharpness is a good sign. After awhile, in a different room of the correct B unit, I retrieve her belongings from the first room and await the interpretation of the test results.

Later, after several more chapters of reading *The Cat Who...* and a shift change, a different ER doctor informs us, "The tests are not pinpointing a problem, so I will admit you to the hospital. Sorry about that, with Christmas Eve almost here." You'll be taken to Unit C to wait until a bed is available. Don't worry. It is a ward; there is a nurse there, and a doctor will drop by from time to time or be called if needed."

Back to purgatory, I think. We'll be reading and waiting on Christmas Eve, but we're together. Again a transport person is called, and we are moved seventy-five feet. I call Karen and Donna to let them know we will not be hosting dinner on the morrow. They are to make their own plans.

Just after the noon hour, I become concerned that my diabetic wife needs some food, but before long a frozen dinner arrives. The afternoon passed with more, *The Cat Who...* Then evening arrives. There are Christmas carols in the ward, which is partitioned with curtains.

We settle in for a longer wait. We don't believe hospitals dismiss patients mid-evening in the dark to make rooms available for others. "We might be in this ward all night," I tell Jacquie. I am almost right.

"Like a lady needing a room two thousand years ago there is not room," Self whispers. The call comes at eleven forty five. She is installed in a special room almost on Christmas morning.

Her room door has a No Exit sign on it. Now what, I wonder. It is an isolation room and quite different from other hospital rooms. I learn that a person goes through a second small room to leave. There is a negative air pressure in this room and it has its own air system and filters. It is the type of room the highly contagious patients were being placed in during the anthrax scare on the East Coast following the New York World Trade Center disaster. Jacquie doesn't have a contagious condition, but like 2001 years ago this evening, it is the only room available to a lady in distress.

Her nurse from the waiting ward accompanies us to the new room and introduces us to her friend, the new nurse for my Jacquie. I kiss Jacquie "Good morning and Merry Christmas," and leave to go home fifteen minutes into Christmas morning. I have not eaten since the cup of coffee and a half banana for breakfast, as the hospital cafeteria closed early for the holiday. Before going to the car, I check the vending machines, but the coin machines are out of sandwiches, and the other machines won't accept dollar bills this evening. On the way home I look for anyplace that is open and serving food, but to no avail. It is go home and fix my own.

I left a box of chocolates for Jane when we left for the hospital. As I turned on the lights I see an envelope on the table for "Jacquie, Don, Mocha and Latte." The card inside is signed, "Jane, Alice and Joe," her dog and cat.

Will JJL being in the hospital lower or increase my stress? Knowing she will have good care is comforting. I go to bed remembering JJL's room number so I won't have trouble finding her. Then I remember that might not hold true. She was switched to another room in the night last July. Will I find her in 3024? Earlier comforting thoughts disappear as I remember, we still don't know what keeps causing her problems, my ongoing worry. Perhaps we have reached the time where we can no longer live together. I notice Self doesn't argue with me as he usually does when I have doubts. I am tired and confused. How much more or longer can we cope? Will I find her in 3024 later this morning this Christmas morning?

After a minimal amount of sleep and with cats and birds fed and watered I shave before eating some cold cereal topped off with strong coffee, I check my gas and head for the hospital. Traffic is reasonable and I'm soon parked and stepping from the elevator onto the third floor and notice my pace hastens as I begin winding my through the corridors and around corners. Room 3024, she's behind the No Exit door and smiling.

"Merry Christmas, Jacquie!" My ill wife of yesterday seems to be quite well today. She is sitting up and quickly holds out her arms and greets me with the same salutation. Since it is an isolation room it is apart from other rooms. She has a large window looking down into a courtyard. We have both slept well and I tell her of my cell calls to the families as I walked into the hospital. I begin reading again to her.

Not long after a nurse says, "Doctor G is our doctor today and he is on the floor now. He will be in to see you soon." This doctor is new to us but he makes a favorable impression in a few minutes.

After listening to her lungs and checking blood pressure, he announces, "Things appear fine this morning. I want to transfer you to another room when one becomes available and if another test or two are normal, I'll dismiss you tomorrow." He then reaches under his left arm and takes her file of records. It becomes apparent he took time before coming to Jacquie's room to study the file contents. "You have had a number of work-ups here with no conclusive result other than probability of having several small TIAs, or minor strokes. The problems they cause are not reversible. I think it is time for you to consider a rest home. Then this gentle giant looked at me and it was apparent his preparation for this conversation had been done, "Mr. Larsen, I find you have suffered from the stress of care taking several times."

I dodge his reference to me and tell him, "Several doctors have on previous visits suggested I consider putting her into a rest home. I think we should consider it seriously," I said.

Before I could turn to Jacquie she chimed it, "Yes, Doctor. I can see what it is doing to Don."

Doctor G answers, "I concur. I will send our dismissal nurse to counsel you as she will be here this morning before going to spend the rest of the holiday with family." The doctor primed her I believe, and after finding I could get some more in-house care from Jane, our housekeeper, the nurse suggests we do that while taking time to look for a rest home. She gives us several pages of guidelines, including a list of agencies and individuals that help locate a rest home suitable to a patient's needs.

The problem is that Jacquie has a good day now and then. Whether she has a good day or not doesn't seem to help my stress level, as I know her spells come and go. I want to wait until her head heals sufficiently to have her eyes checked and get new glasses so she can read. If she will have a roommate who doesn't like all-day TV, JJL may have to return to more reading.

I figure she will be transferred out of the isolation room as soon as another room becomes available, and this happens later on Christmas Day. Her roommate in the new room is a retired teacher by the name of Jacqueline, which is JJL's christening moniker, as well as the name of their nurse. The next morning, the twenty-sixth, I am interrupted in my reading of *The Cat Who...* to my Jacquie when the other asks loudly, "How long is this going to keep up? I didn't get any sleep last night." I stop reading and wink at my Jacquie. The roommate Jacquie doesn't catch up on her sleep that afternoon either as her lunch is served in a few minutes, to be followed by a nurse wanting a blood test. A little later the sleepless Jacquie's catheter becomes a problem and it takes several sessions to remove it and get her settled. "If you remove the catheter and I have no luck, what'll we do then?" she questions the nurse loudly. I almost state just as loudly that I am napping and please quiet down.

"I'll put it back in again," the nurse reassures her.

It is then that I appreciate my Jacquie even more. I certainly don't have the worst behaved Jacqueline in Northern California! The other Jacquie's daughter, or lawyer, arrives to take up much of the rest of the day talking and discussing her moving into a recovery rest home near San Jose. The lady had been there several years ago when she had suffered another stroke. She isn't getting her sleep now that I am quiet.

It is now time for a nice lunch by hospital standards. It wasn't a Christmas dinner she would get at a restaurant but there was a bit of cranberry, a small slice of turkey and a bit of dressing. There is more complaining. "I hope it is better than this morning's oatmeal. That stuff tasted worse than paste!" the roommate states rather pointedly. My Jacquie tells me that the nurse suggested, "Put the milk on the oatmeal," but to no avail. This unhappy woman has a voice as caustic and loud as her temperament. She had been a teacher and as a retired principal, I am glad she is retired and had never been in my school. Kids have enough trouble learning without a cranky and caustic teacher showing them the way.

It's later afternoon and I realize I am tired, so I come home and fall asleep as the five o-clock news is starting. I am luckier than my wife's roommate. I fall asleep. Mel came to visit her grandmother the next day. As she walks into the room, the cranky Jacquie says to her, "I hope you don't visit. I didn't get any sleep last night. The lady you are going to visit snored all night."

Mel is surprised, but not cowed. She replies, "You should have called a nurse and asked for a sleeping pill," and then she went on to say, "Hi Grandma!" Between Mel's visiting and my Jacquie's snoring, the woman become more disgusted that evening and she gets herself moved to another room.

The next roommate makes no noises other than a few groans. She is almost in a coma.

We are preparing to come home on the twenty-seventh, when problems start again for JJL. Coming out of the bathroom, I almost lose my grip on her as she falls forward, and nearly runs across the room out of balance. Later she has another problem, and housekeeping has to be called. It becomes apparent we will need to increase my help at home soon and also find a rest home. More stress for me? We arrive in Livermore without finding why she had pain in her mid-section for four days, but she is feeling better.

Now it is Sunday, the thirtieth and I get ready to host the postponed holiday dinner and gift exchange. Before I start the preparations, I decide to relax with the Sunday paper. It does not take long to read the Sunday paper, but I have trouble reading it. I like to sit on the floor with my feet in the conversation pit and the paper spread flat on the living room floor. Mocha strolls onto it and lies down to stretch across both pages. My attractive and loving feline! Her disruption of my reading is stressing. I find myself reaching out to pet her. As I smile, stroke her soft coat and hear her purr as she looks up at me with an apparent smile, I decide she is also a stress reliever.

"She's like the Chinese sweet and sour combination, Don, a contradiction of actions," Self says rather proud of himself.

I finish the paper later and remove the plastic wrapping from the turkey on the counter. "I'll wait until JJL is awake to salt it inside and out," I tell Self, "so she will feel involved." I am in for a surprise.

When I help her from bed and ask about the salting, she replies, "You must police the cat pan with company coming soon. What time is dinner?'

"One. Now, about the salting."

"You've got to get that pan cleaned. Hurry!"

"I can take care of the pan and a lot of other things once the turkey is in the oven."

"No! Do the pan or I'll do it!" Since with her dizziness she is not to bend over, I change my plans. I'll learn about salting later. The cat pan is policed. JJL starts to move some things off a counter, which I was going to do after the salting. I am beginning to worry about having enough cooking time, but salting does finally occur. "Now take out the middle oven rack so the lower rack is available," I am instructed.

"I've already done that," I inform her.

As she puts the salt container back in the cabinet, and I am picking up the roaster, she reminds me to, "Change the racks to make room for the roaster." Her memory is blinking. I silently hope the morning will improve.

Self, reading my mind, sends his agreement. "Let's not have another 911 and another postponed dinner."

Mel arrives soon, and a little later Karen follows with her contributions for the meal. The morning is off to a fine start. While they take over cooking, I dress Jacquie, and she eases back on her worries and activities. We will have a good Christmas meal on December the thirtieth after all.

But will we make it through the several weeks it will take to clear the paperwork and get her settled into her new home?

"Cross your fingers, Don," is Self's encouragement.

Part Two
Now We Part

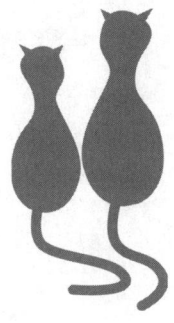

Chapter 26

We Must Leave Each Other
Today's The Day!

Today's the day. I should be ready for it, but I must have had several subconscious concerns, as I awakened at 4:77 this morning. Well, it looked like 4:77 with my glasses off. Some folks make a seven with a line drawn through their downward strokes and that's what I saw on the clock. Still in bed, I put on my glasses and that doesn't make any difference. It's not the fault of the eyes or glasses. The digital clock with the large lighted numerals sits on top of our closet so I can see it in the dark from the bed. Jane must have pushed it back from the edge of the closet top when she cleaned yesterday. As a result, I'm not able to see the bottom lines of the numerals. It is really 4:33. I am now fully awake.

It is to be a busy day. I will attend the first of nearly one hundred real estate marketing meetings I will go to this year to greet Realtors and hand out the word search puzzles I make. I don't charge the company for this time, for several reasons. The three meetings I attend each week are my only social times other than the senior writing class on Tuesday afternoon. Secondly, the company helps us by funding health insurance for Jacquie and me, a valuable benefit this year.

The meeting will be at eight AM in Walnut Creek, in the next county. I normally leave prior to seven, but this morning I need gas, so I will leave even earlier than usual. After the meetings' flag salute that starts the program, I will head home, as I'm not interested in learning about the houses being promoted. Today I must stop by the pharmacy for prescription refills. I should arrive home before Jacquie's medicine wears off and she awakens.

Then, I'll get our breakfast and help her dress. We'll be ready for the day with mixed feelings and anxieties.

This is the day we'll select a rest home for her. It is hard to contemplate separating after fifty-four and a half years of living together after a four-year courtship. At our age we should have monthly marriage anniversaries!

Looking toward this day has not been easy. Several doctors told us she needs to be in a home. At her hospital follow-up appointment the first week of January, Dr. Banda, a soft-spoken lady, looked sternly at us and scolded us for not having her in a home already. To my wife she said, "You have fallen a number of times. You are going to break something in a fall, and then there will be a lot of trouble for everybody, including me." To me, she declared, "The kind of care she needs is more than you can give. It is telling on you! You will both be better off. Do it and do it now!" She said that just like a practicing wife or an administrative judge.

Selfishly, I remember how tired I have been lately, and secretly agree with her. I awakened shortly after midnight yesterday, and had to take a sleeping pill to relax and obtain at least part of my quota of rest. Not good!

Several days ago I interviewed several rest home consultants on the list the dismissal nurse gave us, and I selected Lori, who is coming today to take us to visit five homes in Livermore. She will arrive about eleven so she we can see the homes in their noontime operation. Lori and I spent time on the phone discussing JJL's needs and health requirements. As our cats are a major part of Jacquie's life, I asked about the possibility of taking one with her. Lori said she didn't know about that, but would ask. She has lined up homes to visit that she thinks will best meet JJL's needs. Hopefully, the process will work properly and give a smooth and orderly transition for us.

Penny, our insurance agent and long-time friend, had to find a rest home for her father in a hurry, as he fell and broke a bone or two. She was forced to take the first room available. It wasn't a good choice. Penny gave us the name of a state agency that keeps track of reports on how well rest homes measure to state inspections. We are getting valuable first hand assistance from her that wasn't listed in our policy.

Through the window of my studio I see that the morning star has risen over Mr. Black's rooftop, meaning the sunrise is near. I eat a banana and would like another. I wonder if they are fattening. "Have you ever seen a fat monkey?" Self asks. I'm ready to peel another banana but then get a mental picture of the big belly of an old male orangutan so I decide to skip it. I need to dress and awaken JJL for a quick bathroom visit before putting her to sleep again before I leave.

Puzzles in hand, I leave for the filling station. With a full tank, I head down the freeway on-ramp and meld into the four ribbons of red lights heading westward. For someone who rode the one-row cultivator behind mules in Kansas as a boy, I have adjusted to California's freeways without too much difficulty. I arrived in California before the freeways were very crowded. I used to drive sixty-five mph in the fast left lane if I was in a hurry, and I could pass everyone. Now I drive mostly in the right lane, and even when I'm doing seventy nearly everybody passes me. My job this morning is to watch the taillights of the three cars ahead. If I see a brake light flash up there, I can start to slow.

My driving pattern is automatic, and I begin to realize I'm somewhat tired. In fact, I'm tired all over, including my mind. I am an upbeat person, but lately I've trouble finding any beat. I still take my three-mile walks to stay physically fit, but yesterday it took me all morning to recover. I believe my subconscious mind is stressed and I need to pay attention. I need to do my roll breathing exercises and muscle stretching. In fact, I can do them while driving. For the next five miles I do the exercises and relax a little.

"You need to have some positive thoughts, Don," Self admonishes.

"What's positive?" I try to think of positive things. We don't get the predicted fog, so driving is safer; that's positive "What else is a happy thought?" I ask aloud. My Jacquie has been feeling better lately. That is good and positive news. I realize she worries about the strain she is to me. She is quite thankful for my assistance to her needs. If I go to sleep during an evening TV program, she now lets me sleep, knowing I need to relax, whereas in the past she wakened me, disgusted that I couldn't stay awake. That change is another positive factor.

Another good thought is that there are vacancies currently in local rest homes. We won't have to be on a waiting list for months or find one in another town. What I need is to be able to tell myself to shout Hallelujah! I'll shout it now and often. "Think positive, Don," Self reminds me, "and celebrate all the positive thoughts you can find. Positive thoughts can have curative effects." The fact we took out insurance to help at this time is a big, Hallelujah! I yell Hallelujah loudly three more times and I don't care if the drivers on either side see me yelling to myself. They might think the stock market is up.

I remember how relaxing it is to sit in the rocker in the dark and pet Mocha while taking a break from the computer. Stress seems to flow out my fingers. "Hallelujah!" As I write at the word processor, my mind enjoys the creative process. I scream the H word again! Sharing my writing at class is a positive experience, another H. It is an interesting class of older, positive ... well what should I call them? My class is all females except for me. I probably shouldn't call them old ladies or seniors, but I can definitely say they are all past menopause. They are doing what ex-President Carter suggested in his book, *The Virtues of Aging*, expanding their horizons.

Only a few days before reading his book, I compared my third trimester of life to my first. My thoughts parallel his. Yes, I stubbed my toes and shed tears in each of the trimesters of life, but I also had happy surprises as well. There were opportunities to grow, improve, expand horizons and share in all trimesters. It's up to me to do it and that is Carter's message as well. "Hallelujah for a daughter who gives me meaningful books!"

"Wow, your freeway commute is ending. Rudgear Road exit is just ahead. You'll be at the meeting place with quite a few minutes to spare," my invisible partner notes.

While I wait for the Realtors to arrive I have a pad with me, so I'll jot down a few questions to ask as we visit the potential rest homes for Jacquie in a few hours. But first I need to do some more exercises to lessen what stress is left and hunt for even more positive thoughts. Here's a positive thought – finding out after my ambulance trip six months ago that my sharp pain was not a cardiac pain, but rather is one of stress. Another uplift occurs as I think of the handshakes and hugs I'll share with Realtor friends in a few minutes. Those activities will be especially appreciated this morning.

"Good Morning, Don. How are you?" I'm asked as a hand is extended.

"I'm as well as you look, tremendous!" I reply. I've noticed over the years that most people who ask that question are not really tuned into a response. I intend for them to listen to my answer, so I surprise them. "At my age, any time you see me you know I'm doing great!" is another one I often use. Their eyes fix for a second as they consider what they hear, and then a smile comes to their face. We both relax; I like that.

"I never thought of it that way, Don, but it applies to me too," they answer with a smile that is genuine. I enjoy causing smiles and perhaps that is the reason many people's faces light up when they see me. But maybe they are laughing at an old fool with an odd face.

When the meeting starts, I head out the side door quietly and then start home to help JJL get ready for her day. After the finger pricking for blood sugar testing and her insulin shot, I start to help her from bed. She resists, announcing; "I don't feel good enough to go looking at rest homes. You go without me." She looks as ill as she says she feels, but I tell her she needs to get dressed anyhow, as Jane is coming to clean house. I give her the many pills required and get breakfast for us.

Then it is time to get dressed. I'll get her slacks on straight this morning. That is important, and it has taken me several days and admonishments to learn to do it right. I once threatened to take her to a tattoo parlor to have a centerline tattooed on her belly so I could have a guideline. We'll be ready for the day with mixed feelings and anxieties.

We are ready for Lori a few minutes early and as we seat ourselves in our double recliner Latte jumps to JJL's lap and Self asks for my attention. "Don, I'm reminded of the late evening before a big wedding. The atmosphere is heavy with the anxieties, worries, hopes, fears and second-guessing of mother and daughter. Both want a successful conclusion but apprehension in the backs of their minds. While JJL is rather down you will side with Lori whose business is to be upbeat. However, Don, I sense deep down you feel you might be betraying your Jacquie. Right?"

"It is a big step and I have troubled feelings. I know we're probably doin' the right thing, but frankly, I'm finding it hard to do. Since we've or I've gotta' do it, I want to do it in a way that doesn't cause feelings to run deeper, if you know what I mean."

"Remember, You have a lot going for you. That is positive, don't forget it."

"Such as…"

"You picked Lori, someone who knows her business, to help you. You feel good about your conversation with her. Remember you noticed she was a good listener. She knows of at least five openings in town and she knows the homes and the owners. You don't have to take only what is available as did your friend Penny. That place she had to accept for her dad didn't work out and he died soon after arriving. She had a right to have bad internal feelings, you don't even have to take any of the five you are to see today. Buck up, Don. Jacquie's counting on you. Don't talk too much and look and listen a lot. Good luck!"

I had just leaned back and was considering Self's remarks when the doorbell rang.

"She's here. Get the door, Don," my wife commands. "I don't feel like going anywhere."

As I open the door, the lady standing there and I exchange smiles as she asks, "Mr. Larsen?" and to my nod she announces, I'm Lori." This nice but simply attired lady spots Jacquie and walks to the recliner to introduce herself. "I'm Lori. I met Don by phone and know about your basic needs. I'm early and would like to become acquainted with you before we start our visits."

Self has been with me in evaluating a lot of teachers and other employees acts as if it is he who will further evaluate Lori. "This lady looks pretty average but she certainly acts like a professional should, allowing time to get acquainted and demonstrating genuine interest. I'm impressed."

It is immediately apparent this lady is at home helping people find new quarters. Her manner is one of listening with understanding as does Self. "Don, I notice Jacquie is perking up and becoming more at ease. Her answers and conversation with Lori are sincere and beginning to show confidence. Take that to heart, Don. Those are great signs."

I don't know if her breakfast helped or whether the positive Lori affects her but JJL appears to feel better. After a few minutes of getting acquainted, we are off to visit five homes.

We go first to a group of five houses on one lot six blocks from home. While our guide is polite and the grounds and quarters clean, we are not impressed. The owner meets us for only a moment and leaves. He and his establishment seem to be more geared to a facility than to a caring home. While we were shown all five houses we were not shown the empty rooms available to JJL. We left.

In the west part of town we find a nice house that gave the feeling of a caring home. My instant opinion was, it'll do, if we don't find anything better. The available room was nice but quite small. It was a front bedroom beside the recessed entry. Jacquie suffers diarrhea far too often and the long walk the length of the entry to a long hall to a bathroom was a serious detriment. "Let's see the other homes," I inform Lori while JJL remained non-committal.

The fifth house and site were quite attractive and only three miles northeast from our house. The door opened to Lori's touch to the doorbell button and we were greeted to an interesting sight. Beyond the tiny but open entryway was the dining room with housemates at lunch. Several smiling Filipino ladies were turned to face us. I noted that the smiles were of the genuine variety and loaded with feeling. I was beginning to be impressed. The lady opening the door offered me her hand and said, "I'm Maribec, the owner. Welcome to Chateau Livermore. You must be Mr. Larsen,' and turning to Jacquie, "And you are Mrs. Larsen. Welcome. While the ladies are eating, let me show you our home," and she moved to the family room with its six recliners and large TV set.

"Maribec is a nurse," Lori said to JJL. She and her husband own six or seven homes and and has been in the care industry for seventeen years. It is a full time job for her. I've known her several years. She runs a good home. Maribec, why don't you show the Larsens your empty room." We were led down a hall past bedrooms and a common bath to the room designed as a master bedroom where our hostess indicated the available bed with her left hand. This was a large room with a big picture window overlooking a nice rear yard. There was a second single bed beside a large master bathroom. JJL and I went into this room. It had a large tub with handles removed and an oversized shower equipped for drizzles with a chair and nozzle on a hose. While JJL wasn't well she didn't miss the apple tree outside the large window or the amount of light from the giant skylight.

"Don," Self whispered, "I know you would like to stay to study the home more but I note Jacquie is tiring fast."

To Maribec and Lori, I said, "I think Jacquie needs to get to bed and rest. I like what I see but want to talk to my wife a bit before we decide. Maribec, will you hold the room twenty-four hours for us. I'll call tomorrow. I need to make one more check with our insurance company. They had a nurse examine Jacquie a week ago and we should have their answer today. Thanks again, Maribec."

We head home and rest. After Lori leaves and after Jacquie's nap, we talk. "They were warm smilers who made me feel comfortable right away," I reminded JJL. "You can have your own TV and phone, so you will feel less institutionalized. Your roommate is almost deaf and blind so she won't be a talker. Lori will make the paperwork arrangements."

"What's her fee for helping us?"

"She'll collect her finder fee from the rest home owner we chose."

While the several hour tour has been physically tiring to my Jacquie it is also quite stressful to me planning our separation after fifty-four and a half years of living together. I go to the computer for some Solitaire to help me relax. I'm not sure it is relaxing to choose a card only to have Mocha stand in front of the screen to watch my arrow move and block that part of the screen from my view. I move her a bit, but that large, bushy tail still hides the cursor. She loves me, I will appreciate that affection as Jacquie, my love of fifty-four and a half years, moves to another residence. Neither Mocha or solitaire relax me, so I lie down beside my JJL.

Later in the day I read the agreement of conditions and rules of what may be JJL's new home. We decide this home will meet our needs. I call Penny to check on the insurance company's actions. She also gives me the name of an a state agency that monitors rest homes. I call the agency and the officer in charge checks the file with history of their inspections of the Chateau. There are two entries. One is a note that a window screen was not completely fastened in place. The other was also a non-issue. We decide JJL will accept the Chateau as her new home. I call Lori and Maribec with the decision.

I begin to fill our pillboxes for the next week. I put my pillboxes back into the cabinet, but leave JJL's on the table to take with her to her new Chateau Livermore residence when the paperwork is finished. Leaving the evidence of the move in sight helps us both with the reality of the change in our lives. From time to time in the next few days we will think of items to pack for the move: a small clock, pen and pencil, tweezers, and the like. The move is settling into our consciousness.

After dinner JJL turns to her favorite TV program and I decide to stretch out for a few minutes on the bed. It has been a long day. In fact, it has been fourteen hours since I rose at 4:77 AM. I wonder if a soak in a tub of hot water will relax me further. That thought leads to a catastrophe. I should have seen it coming. I didn't!

We bought a cast iron tub when we built the house, and hung it through the bedroom floor next to the lavatory cabinet. Since it is iron and hangs into the cold crawl space below the floor, the first bath water cools rather quickly in the winter. Tonight I run three inches of hot water only to warm the tub, intending to fill it later when I'm ready to soak. I undress except for my wedding ring and go to the little toilet room while the tub is heating. I received a book at Christmas to help people learn more history while in the bathroom. I am reading about Cleopatra when the catastrophe occurs.

This month there is an airline commercial that asks, "Has there been a time..." and it proceeds to show a situation. In this week's version a guest opens the hostess's medicine cabinet. The top glass shelf breaks and, with everything on it falls to break the glass shelves below. The cascade continues through all the shelves into the basin below, with sounds of breaking glass and crashing. Then the commercial's voice continues "... when you need to get away in a hurry?" and a plane climbs into the sky. What I hear is just such a sound of crashing glass.

I wonder if JJL has fallen but the noise is wrong; she hits things with a thud when she falls. There is no glass near her. Before I can call out, "Are you OK?" she shouts the same thing to me. We then know that the other is fine and the noise is somewhere between us. Wearing only my ring, I head into the dark master bedroom. Latte is sitting in the ten-foot-wide doorway between the bedroom and the dining room, rather unconcerned. Mocha is six feet farther away in the dining room, and she appears OK also. But wait, her fluffy tail is less fluffy near the end.

It is dark outside, and the neighbors could see into the dining room through the glass walls of my studio, so I call to Jacquie, "I'll get my pants on and check Mocha. She appears to have wet spots." I pick up the towel beside the tub and soon have her feet and the end of her tail dry. She must have jumped into the tub looking for a spider or expecting me to play a catch game with a paper I often wave over the tub edge. Since the bedroom is dark she could not see the water. The noise we heard was a lot of frantic kicking, splashing and scratching as she tried to make for a quick getaway from her surprise foot bath. I run more water and have a good soak and several chuckles. It is a good stress reliever!

Now that we have chosen the rest home, we are at ease with the fact that we need it. That worry is past. It is not so for two of our three children. Larry, our son in Kansas, is used to dealing with the aged as an EMT, so he is more accepting. A day after being told of our decision, Karen tells us we are more settled with her mother's move than she and Jon. After being reminded how we had to bring JJL's mother into our home and how Darrel's grandmother had failed. Karen reconciled herself to the facts.

Jon took it harder. "Dad, Mom can fall in a rest home just as accidentally as she can at home," Jon tells me. I agree, and we talk some more. He slowly realized the stress is on both of us as we now function. It's as hard for children to accept some facts of life as it is for a spouse. I set it up so Jon can help me choose a new TV for her Saturday, and that seems to help. He volunteers his son, Drew, to help move the luggage, and that seems to help everyone.

Jon is our youngest and a lot like his mother: rather quiet and like her has a shy smile. He was a baby when we arrived in the Golden State. He was not a problem as a child except for one day in the sixth grade. I had just accepted the principal-ship at his school when the teacher sent another boy to my office for discipline. It was stuffy in the my small office and the boy drew himself into the military attention mode before saying, "There's another boy in this, Sir!"

"Who's that?" I demanded.

"Your son, Sir."

I called the room and told the teacher, "Send Jon to the office." The boys were playing cards under desks and chairs they pushed into a corner for cover. I called JJL and told her Jon was on his way home. As I was talking to the other parents I had to interrupt, "Oops, your son is fainting." When he came to he was on my lap looking up at my face while Jon was holding the boys legs high so blood could drain back to the head. The nurse was fanning him. The boys were never sent to me during the rest of the year.

It appeared that Jon wasn't going to be the student he could be. As JJL and I were soon to be by ourselves the house the two older children had helped us build two decades earlier was going to be too big for us. It was time for down sizing and also time to show Jon how to use his hands. It might help him choose a trade. Once we had a lot we determined the floor plan and he drew it as part of a high school project. We finished it but Jon wanted to be a mechanic. He married Donna a week or two before school was out and they moved to Denver for a year of schooling. As he wanted to be a diesel mechanic he studied harder than ever before to be in the top of the class for acceptance for a semester of diesel training.

He became a Caterpillar employee for several years before solvents in oils kept his hands checked and cracked. This forced him to quit. It was then he came to work at the house inspection company I started. He became operations manager while Donna served as office manager and Jacquie was chief editor and company secretary. Now Jon and Donna run the company with me doing the marketing.

The new home and our family are ready, but JJL can't move until some paperwork is completed. Lori faxed a medical report form to our doctor, but after several days of waiting, it hasn't been returned. Lori asks me if I can help. I have to go for a prescription so I check with a nurse. "The paperwork probably went to the business office," she tells me. We retrieve the form and after it has been completed and reviewed, sign it. Another Hallelujah! Jacquie can move.

It's the eventful afternoon. We pack her clothes, medicines and after looking around the house and petting each of the cats she turns to the garage to leave. Picking up Drew we drive to the Chateau. . I have prepared a sheet of Jacquie's problems and other things the caretakers should know. I am pleased with the care and time taken by the lady in charge to go over the facts. Her name is Susan. She is a listener, and I like people with authority who listen to what others have to say. I will learn a lot more about Sue before long. With unpacking done we step to the little porch outside her room and enjoy the flowers the view she'll have from her window. My wife is now installed, and we will sleep at two different addresses after fifty-four and a half years. "I'll see you tomorrow," I tell her as I kiss her good-bye. But before I take the long three strides to the hallway to leave her, I turn and announce, "I need one more good hug to last me till tomorrow. We enjoy several meaningful moments before I turn and walk. It is January the seventeenth.

That night both cats look for their Jacquie's lap but decide it is OK to sleep on mine since the mistress is not around. I notice that Mocha takes a detour some distance from the tub as she follows me to the bathroom.

It is Saturday and Jon and I buy a small TV for Jacquie's use. I let him talk me into a more expensive set for her. When I said I would get earphones for her and run a wire over the door and beside the bed, he suggested cordless earphones. She can listen to TV without disturbing her roommate. JJL and I appreciated his suggestion. We get a set of nice earphones. JJL's move has gone smoothly. Self says, "Don, I believe she had almost looked forward to it. She was very concerned about your health. I heard her tell Jon, your dad looks tired. I'm so sorry he has to work so hard and long to care for me. That is a statement of love, Don." Hearing doctors tell her it was time to seek extra help readied her subconscious mind.

"Our preparing for the move over several days helped as did Lori's friendliness and good words about the home. Lori promised to stop by the Chateau to check on Jacquie several times in the next weeks.

Our friend Dodo's mother has fallen and broken two shoulders in the last year, and it is more than Dodo can handle. Now single and in her seventies she runs a craft store. To make matters worse, the mother is in her nineties and too proud to go to a home. Dodo is closing her store in a month, but she looks so tired and stressed, I wonder if she herself will last that long. We are lucky that Jacquie is so accepting of the move. The support and help of Jon, Karen and Drew are important factors also, I believe.

Chapter 27

End Of A Part Of Our Life
JJL And I Start Over

In the very young years, a child wants to be a fireman, policeman, cowboy or something else. Later, in high school, this first decision is revamped and changed. Choosing a mate is another stage of life, as is raising a family. In time, the family becomes a couple again as the children leave the nest. Other variations can and do occur. This is the week Jacquie and I have ended the "live-together couple" part of our life and, started another life phase. We now need help to live our lives. She starts a phase called Outside Assisted Living. I will be living alone but the cats will solve much of my loneliness.

"Can you handle it OK?" Self asks.

"The real question is, how will we adjust?" I tell him. "Just as we planned the previous parts or stages of our lives, more planning is needed now, I believe. Too many elderly people and their families just allow aging to happen. They do no planning. They just drift through their later years."

"So you're going to be different?" Self says.

"I don't intend for that to happen to us. I need to take a few days to do more planning and then several weeks or months to put the plans into effect," I reply. I have done many of Jimmy Carter's suggestions in *Virtues of Aging.* Now I need to revamp my plans to fit our latest situations.

Jacquie and her short term needs are my first priority. Her health care needs are fairly well met now. Each time I hear a good statement about Chateau Livermore, I share it with her to help her feel better. I have a long visit with her main caregiver last night, and I'll share part of that with Jacquie. Karen, our daughter, suggests her mother needs something manipulative to help with her muscles, and also to pass the time. I agree, but I'm having problems coming up with a solution. JJL liked to play solitaire on her computer, and I could take it to her. She is still thinking about entering all our bills into a bookkeeping program, but she isn't up to that, so I'll leave the computer here until I've mailed our taxes. I looked at the little handheld solitaire games in computer stores, but the buttons may be too confusing. She is having trouble adjusting to her new TV remote buttons. When I ask if she wants a new pack of cards, I'm told, "My hands won't let me shuffle a deck."

I did take her a small jigsaw puzzle, and after she works it, I may take others. She has a magazine of crossword puzzles and I need to replace it when it's finished. The TV, Latte and naps have filled her days for the last year, so maybe she will be OK. Fortunately she is starting to read again, now that the swelling on the head from the fall has disappeared. She received new glasses a week ago but is unable to hold large books so she appreciates the smaller paperbacks.

Part of my short-term plan is to include some walking. There is a ramp to the exterior of the home and on most days we can go for short walks outside. It will be a break for her and a means of keeping her muscles from deteriorating. If we do it together, she will learn to look forward to my visits. It will be a different togetherness. Since the other ladies are in their eighties and nineties, and somewhat infirm, the exercise inside is all but nonexistent. JJL had me make a list of the exercises she is to do and print it on a sheet for her. "Good for my non-exercising wife," I tell Self.

"Yup, those are exercises she can do by herself in bed, Don, or on her couch."

I will also ask her for a lunch or dinner date now and then. The home is accepting of that and will "get her ready for dates," Sue states as she raises her hand for a high-five from me. I like that little woman already.

Susan has become Sue to JJL in only a day or so and Sue has already taken to me as part of her team and feels comfortable telling me what "your Jacquie needs." She greets me with a smile or a giggle some days and a very serious mood others as she talks on a cell phone as she sets the table or sorts the washing. Her short frame appears to be a strong asset as she must help the ladies about in many cases. She handles the care, the housekeeping and the cooking alone. On days when she is not there two ladies replace her.

The cats' psychological health may be a concern, but I go out of my way to notice and love them. I took them to see her several days ago and it worked fine. While the owner of the Chateau said JJL could have a cat, Sue is afraid of them. Besides she opens all doors to air the house and the cats could go out and get lost. She gives good service so I don't want to push her by asking her to care for a cat also. JJL has no business doing cat chores. Skeptically, Sue suggests I continue the cat visits. Several days later, I take the cats for a second visit. A frail lady with only one leg, who hasn't shown any spark of life, turns in her chair when she hears the word cat. Her face lights up with animation, and she is eager to pet Mocha. She loves cats. I guess Mocha may make regular visits.

I go out for breakfast as a gift for myself. I lie on the couch upon returning. Mocha snuggles to me, lets me pet her and then turns to present her other side. This process is repeated for ten minutes. When I put my shoes on she helps me. Latte sleeps beside or upon me, and tells me when it is time for her wet food. I think the felines will adjust to JJL's absence and we will not need an animal psychologist.

I look forward to going to the Chateau to see JJL each day. I've always liked to bring her surprises, and will try to continue to do that at her new home. I can't bring many goodies from the bakery due to diabetes, but there are other things. She has a Jeweler's orchid in bloom, and I can take a spike to her in a vase. Our first camellia blossom opened this morning, and that can be a Sweetie Gift tomorrow. I stop at a store that has pieces of bread pudding. She loves it, and when we cut the large piece into several parts, her diabetes won't suffer too much. This little sharing will continue to go a long way with both of us.

In the week she has been there, I have seen no other family members visiting Jacquie's housemates. Penny, our insurance lady, says that far too many elderly are simply dumped into homes and forgotten. It's not in my plans to forget JJL. I have sent her address to family members, and if we get her a phone I will send the phone number also. She did not use a phone at home, so not having one is not traumatic. This follow-through on my part is helping me get past the separation. Knowing she can call me on my cell phone will be a comfort to both of us.

"Ah, heck Don, get her a cell phone." I thank Self and get her one to match mine.

After I catch up on some postponed work around the house and yard I will tackle the long-term options I would like to pursue. Before I do, I may read Jimmy Carter's *The Virtues of Aging* once more. I will also use the Internet to do more research on ways to enjoy the aging process and get the most satisfaction from it. Probably I will continue to check web sites for more information about small strokes or TIAs that JJL suffered. I may even have lunch with a friend now and then. One suggested it the other day, and I realize I had not done that in years. It would be a step in the healing direction.

My initial search on the Internet turned up some information we had not learned at the HMO facilities:

TIAs, transient ischemic attacks, are often a precursor of a stroke

Any numbness, slurred speech or unusual muscle twitching should be reported to the medical people immediately and seen by them within forty five minutes

Blood clotting for a period of time causes death of brain cells that cannot be re-grown or replaced, hence the permanent damage of a stroke, mini or major in nature

Quick intervention with blood thinners often minimizes or avoids the effects of a stroke. Some effects can be overcome.

There is a lot of other information. Studying it and other topics will be one of my long-term goals.

I awaken this Monday at four. I check my mind and find it is alert and not in need of more sleep. I check my body and don't find it ready for the day. It is content to stay where it is, in bed. I check further. I'm sleeping better than in the past and I've been walking. I've had my usual six hours of rest. The question is whether it is fatigue or whether the feeling is a default setting found in the senior stage of life and associated with arthritis, worn joints and worn-out muscle groups. I believe it is the latter so I'll not try to return the alert mind to sleep. I'll tell the body to use the muscles or lose them.

Today is to be a day of future action planning. I now am caught up with my list of current and emergency items, so I need to project toward the future. I'll carry my little notebook with me and jot down ideas for future actions. Companies often go to a resort or an exotic town to do planning. I can do it without going away. I can do my planning as I lounge in bed, as I drive the freeway to Realtor meetings or as I deliver reports and newsletters. I'll plan!

One top priority, as soon as I get out of bed, is to print my weight on a piece of paper and hang it on the refrigerator. I'm too heavy. I'll also take the dark chocolate sundae-topping jar to the trashcan. I dumped my rich spinach dip last night. Progress!

Today I will package the request for the insurance company to pick up JJL's care. The paperwork is done and ready to send. Putting that into the mail will finish a major task.

During the week I'll have other activities. I'll finish delivering my January inspection newsletter and start writing the February edition. February will feature tips for inspecting new and nearly new houses. I'll work with Jon on that and have an appropriate photo. Another task is to get organized for preparing our income taxes. I'll sort through the accumulation of receipts and cull those of tax value. As time becomes available, I'll start the adding process and draw blank lines for information yet to come in the mail. I want to be as current on preparation as possible so JJL won't worry.

"Don, that won't happen. She'll worry anyhow," Self chides.

Next week I will continue the tax task, and start distributing the February newsletter. I'll then begin to clean the garage, as it's almost full. On my walks, I find many residences where several cars are parked outside, and if the garage door is open, the space inside is crammed with possessions. What's more, huge rental storage units being built all over town. We buy big houses, and yet we accumulate more than they can hold. I don't want that to happen to me. I need to rid our house of some things.

As I tidy the kitchen, I start making some decisions. Decisions are important. Thursday I dropped newsletters in a real estate office in Orinda and was pleased to see the almost elderly lady behind the counter looking so well. She said, "Good morning. I haven't seen you for awhile."

I replied, "I don't market in December, because Realtors are preoccupied with the holidays like everyone else. By the way, you not only look like you are feeling well; you look several years younger than when I saw you in November. I mean it. It's not flattery."

She smiled and said, "Thank you. I've made some difficult decisions and I do feel much better." Before leaving I told her about my favorable opinion of Jimmy Carter's book *The Virtues of Aging*.

"That lady is proof," I tell Self. Making decisions and acting on them has positive effects."

There are a few checks to write, and I begin, but am soon interrupted. Friendly Mocha rubs her head upon the top of my pen, causing my handwriting to vary considerably and make me look like I'm becoming feeble. There's another reason for on-line commerce. Mocha seems to have more love than that little body can hold, and she must share it. "You're lucky, Don. It's Hallelujah time again!" Self is so right!

Staring at the ceiling, I start some decisions about the culling process. First I'll gather things of no use or value to us. I'll ask the kids if they want any of them and after they've made their choices I will decide the fate of the rest. Some items will go to the trash, some I'll donate to a worthy cause, and some will find themselves in a garage sale. The next concern will be those things that may have some family value, for example, my paintings. I've recently stopped entering shows, as I am not producing new paintings. If the kids don't want them, I'll do a special garage sale. The HMO is building a new set of offices in our town and maybe they can use them as a donation. The paint supplies will go into an art garage sale when one of the associations holds one. I'll keep the artwork we display, and let the kids settle that after we're gone. The same rules will hold for furniture: get rid of some and keep the rest. Some furniture goes back three generations. I'll try to have most of this done in six months. I'll not do things that will upset Jacquie when she comes to visit.

As I get up for a coffee break, I smile, and remember the sorting I did yesterday morning. When I pulled open the drawer for a pair of sox, I noted there was a mix-up of pairing. I had the time, so I pulled all the socks from the drawer and matched them with several individual socks on the counter. I then opened JJL's drawer, where I found more of mine. Looking under the sink, I found another pair. There was only one pair of my favorite low white socks, so I will check my wife's drawer for more when I finish this cup. I was going to buy some more socks, but maybe I should look in the refrigerator and piano first. Perhaps I need to talk to Jane.

My mind turns to Jacquie. "How's she doing?" I'll leave to visit her minutes after the socks.

Chapter 28

Together, We Live Apart
By Darn! Let's Make It Work!

How we doing? OK, No, I mean really? Our separate lives seem to be functioning as we had hoped they would. Will it stay that way?

It's two weeks later, and all but one thing is going fine. JJL seems to be happy and looks better. That is the view shared by the family, the caretaker and Lori, the lady who helped us find the home. JJL's face is relaxed, and she seems to have settled into the home and its routine. What more can we ask? The one hitch is a change of time routine. She eats at seven, eleven and four. She is in bed at five or six and lights are out at eight. That is a lot earlier than going to bed after the eleven PM newscast. She doesn't complain, though, if that's the only hitch we have, it's a great placement.

She is having a social life, but it is somewhat narrow. Several of the ladies do no talking. I called Sue and asked for a dinner date. I'm told, "Why not? I'll have her ready."

"I'll pick her up at five."

"I'm not very hungry, Don," Jacquie says when I arrive. "Sue fed me at four. How about just desserts?" We share some bread pudding and enjoy two hours together. I take her into her room at seven. Everyone else is in bed, and JJL's nightdress is laid out for her. I get her ready for bed and after tucking her in, kiss her goodnight. This is the first date of our new life. It's a successful one to boot.

Tuesday I call after cutting out of writing class, to ask Sue, "Did you and Jacquie remember that she has an appointment this afternoon for her haircut? I'm on the way."

"Yes. I'll have her in the wheelchair and by the door. By the way, she told me not to wait dinner as you were going to take her out to eat. Ha, ha." Mentally I could see the twinkle in our Sue's eyes.

"Don," Self asks, "are these women ganging up on you?"

When we start to leave the house I transfer Jacquie to her walker and am holding her arm against falling. Sue gives me a dirty look and insists in a non-arguable tone, "If you take any of my patients on a date, you must use her wheelchair!" I sense JJL not only respects but also appreciates Sue. Then she confides to me, "It bugs me that Sue won't let me move without holding onto me,"

"That's because I told her to do just that!" I inform my wife. I get the wrinkled nose treatment with the stuck out-tongue.

"Why?"

"Because you never know when you will black out or become dizzy, that's why!" I say rather adamantly. "She's doing a good job of following orders just like she can give them. She is a good sergeant."

JJL also has to wear a pullover knitted cap to keep her head warm. "Be careful driving ," I'm told, "you have one of my patients!" I believe we have a serious caretaker.

"What time is curfew?" I ask with a grin.

"Seven prompt," I am informed

As we drive away, I ask if Sue ever takes a day off. "Sue says she loves her job," Jacquie replies

"I think people should like their jobs, or try to find one they do like," I remark. "Life has too much to offer to be stuck in a situation. I think she'll give you better care since she enjoys caring work. Think what it would be if your caretaker didn't like it!"

Sue is an interesting person we are learning. She's the CEO of the site. She's efficient and runs the house like clockwork on her schedule. Arising for her shower at five she proceeds to awaken her charges for undressing and redressing. Jacquie shakes her head as she describes the dressing process. "Yesterday's plastic undergarments are stripped off and new ones installed for our day ahead. Then Sue stretches the garment outward and dumps a handful of baby powder inside, both front and back. She says the proper way to dress is to pull on the slacks before the T-shirt so that's the way it's done. After the T-shirt is on, it too is pulled from us front and back for more handfuls of powder."

"I've noticed all the ladies wear t-shirts,"

"Yes. Sue doesn't have time to button blouses. Next comes a zip up-sweater or a sweatshirt so we elder ladies don't become cold. Before the dressing session, one of us will be given a shower."

"Like the drizzle you had at home, I suppose."

"Yes. After she has us dressed, she opens all the doors and windows to air the house. Sue says, 'That's the way we do it in the Philippines.' I will admit the house doesn't have any of the odors of some care facilities."

"She's as colorful as she is efficient," I observe. "Her denim short-shorts over black panty hose and her sleeveless knit shirts set her apart from other caregivers I've seen."

"In spite of her blustery ways, she is very caring. Yet she can scold us if we don't go by the house rules, her rules. Lately she has been confiding in me. 'Jacquie, I'm going to Hawaii on my next time off. Don't tell anybody, it's a secret between the two of us.' She's usually talking in her native language on a cell phone to friends as she makes her housekeeping rounds, and I'll bet she lets her cat out of the bag before I do."

That portable phone is Sue's constant companion, it seems. In fact, I learn she has two of them and she talks as she works wherever she is sorting the wash or sweeping.

We arrive at the restaurant Jacquie wanted to go to for my birthday. They were to have prime rib and she could have a baked potato with sour cream. We were too full for anything sweet so we drove home in the moonlight. I notice her hand come to rest on my knee as she says, "This was a nice evening, I love you, Don. Thanks for being so good to me."

After a nice dessert another evening, it is time to go to a store for some house slippers and a new supply of disposable undergarments. All the occupants must wear them. JJL again tells me that Susie insists on dressing and undressing the ladies. In my wife's case, that is a good idea, as JJL becomes dizzy as she bends over. The wheelchair makes it relatively easy for us to look at slippers, and we enjoy looking at several other items. Jacquie has not been in a store other than an occasional grocery store in more than a year. She becomes tired, however, and it is time to beat Sue's curfew. This evening causes me to feel like a young man again as JJL wouldn't let me take her into a store for years; it's just like old times but with wheels.

"Any stress now?' Self asks. I wrinkle my nose and stick out my tongue.

After leaving JJL I exit as Sue is sitting on the floor in front of her sound system singing into her cordless microphone. I tell her she acts like a Sergeant. She thinks about my remark for a moment, then breaks out into a fit of laughter. She raises her hand for a high-five. "You're right," she says. "I like that!" She takes it as a sign of respect.

"And I follow your orders," I say, "as if you are a sergeant." Another spell of giggling and another high-five. I could still hear her singing as I entered the car on the other side of the street. Fortunately, her songs are happy ones.

Driving home I smile as I realize how fortunate we are to have found this home. Sue's cooking is different from the mid western variety we were raised on. The Kansas farm diet was rich with gravies, butter and a lot of vegetables. Sue sticks to more of a school cafeteria menu. But JJL can handle the change I believe. "If I need such a home," I said to myself, "I hope I can find a home with a Sue-type sergeant."

Several days later it is nice weather when I stop to see my JJL. I invite her to go with me as I deliver an inspection report to a Realtor in the next county. She is tired and declines.

"Don, I left my purse at the optometrist's office. Would you get it for me the next time you are downtown, please." She didn't miss it earlier as I always pay any charges.

"Sure! No problem." That will be easy I think. One shouldn't make judgment too soon.

The next day is beautiful. There is snow on the hills around our valley, and it comes almost to our green valley floor. We have one of these days every few years. I enjoy the scenery while delivering inspection reports.

As I'm traveling with the seventy-mile-per-hour freeway crowd, I note in my left side view mirror a yellow streak fast catching me. A shiny, hot mustard-colored car speeds by and keeps weaving through the traffic ahead. It still has the paper in the license plate holder to attest to its newness. The lady driver is smartly dressed and sitting quite upright. She has her new convertible's top down despite the forty-degree temperature.

As I grin and shake my head Self remarks, "Is she trying out her heater's top setting or just showing off?"

Before going home, I stop at the optometrist's office for JJL's purse. "My wife left her purse here after her examination last Monday. I'm here to retrieve it." There is a look of surprise, which tips me off to a setback.

"We have no extra purses," one of the bevy of ladies informs me.

"Are you insinuating that you did a good job of cleaning each night, and that I had better check the car for it or clean my house?" I say with a raised eyebrow and a grin before I leave.

I stop at the Chateau to see Jacquie and tell her, "You didn't leave the purse at the eye doctor's office."

"I did. I left it beside the big mirror the lady brought to the trying-on table. Ask them again, Don," she says as I leave.

Self observes, "Don, you're in a tight spot. Did she leave it?" I shrug a shoulder and vow to keep on checking.

Each day has its own beginning. Now that it is becoming light outside this morning, I need to feed the birds. Yesterday I put a number of peanuts in the feeders, hoping the squirrels living to the south would smell them. Coming into the studio, I find the neighborhood blue jays have found the nuts and quickly and efficiently are removing them. These fellows are professional scrappers. The other birds scatter at the sight of blue in the distance, but it doesn't stop there. The jays bluff and scrap with each other. They are saucy, scrappy, arrogant, colorful, clownish and rude. There were five of them yesterday, and they put on quite a show. When the peanuts are gone, the jays disappear also. I don't mind, as the other birds wait in the wings and are soon feeding rather peacefully.

I have received word that the HMO in San Francisco wants to include me in a follow-up study of bypass patients of several years ago, which means going to have an EKG. I have agreed to it, and since I don't like to drive in the city, I have elected to go by rapid transit. When I awoke, I didn't know it would be a day of frustration, which I would be glad to see end.

Before the day starts I called about the purse once more. "Hello. Have you found Mrs. Larsen's purse? Remember, I may not pay for her glasses if you don't find the purse." No purse!

"Don, do you suppose one of the employees took her purse?" Self implores. "I don't remember it. Could your JJL be wrong. I'd hate to see you make a goat of yourself." I shake my head and shrug my shoulders as I'm beginning to wonder also.

There are five reports to be delivered to four cities. The last one is near a BART station. Bay Area Rapid Transit handles a lot of people. In fact, it handles more passengers than it has car parking. That is almost where the trouble starts. One nice realty office lady I hand a report to suggests that I go to the large grocery and buy senior Bart tickets to save some money. Due to some labor problem, they are out of tickets: No big problem, since I hadn't known about the discount when I made my decision to travel by Bart. I enter the parking lot and find only one spot in the two large lots. I park in it. As I reach the steps to the loading platform, I see a sign stating stall numbers relate to an occupant's number. I mistakenly assume that the number means the spot is a reserved one and I can't park there. I find later, it's only a number to help remember which stall you parked in. I go another ten miles to the west to the next station. I find a lot of ONE WAY ONLY and EXIT ONLY signs, but finally enter the parking lot, to find it full also. I ask the transit police officer, "How does one find a parking spot?"

"Just wait until a train comes and someone gets off. Go then to their spot." I park and turn the radio to some nice classical music. Sure enough a lady gets off, but she walks out of the lot and to a home nearby.

I approach the officer again and he sees our blue handicapped sign. "Park in a handicapped spot and hang your tag," he says with the smile that says he knows he is helping. I drive to that area but those spots are filled also. As I drive by him again, he waves me down. "Try the other lot, it's bigger." It, too, is full.

I look for a freeway on-ramp and find I'm trapped in a narrow street. A huge semi truck is trying to back up to the rear of a small grocery store. The front of the truck blocks the street ahead, and several cars have followed me onto the street, preventing me from backing out. I begin to wonder if I will make it to HMO in time for my EKG. I think I'll have time if my drive to San Francisco goes OK, I tell myself, as I finally ease onto the elevated freeway. The city looks clean and bright across the bay and I'll soon be there. After I cross the Bay Bridge, I drop from the freeway onto the ground-level streets, and I begin to wonder where Geary Boulevard is. It has been a decade or so since I've driven in the city. I find the street, but my troubles began all over again. Since it is a thoroughfare I can't make a left turn. Passing the hospital, I started making right turns to be able to cross Geary at a signal. I might have expected it. There are a lot of courts, cul-de-sacs and dead ends on the top of that hill, a few hundred feet from the hospital. In time, I am beside the building I want, but I can't find parking.

"Again, everything's against you," Self mutters. I would be in time if I could just park. A sign appears with an arrow directing me to a building two blocks away. Parking on the fifth level, I begin to stretch my tired legs with a walk up one of San Francisco's hills. I left home at a little before ten, and thought I would arrive with a lot of time to have a cup of coffee and perhaps a short walk to take in the view. It's a good thing I started early, as I arrive at 2:25, only five minutes ahead of my appointment.

The EKG goes fine and Self wonders, "Why did you spend half a day getting to the city for a fifteen-minute test?"

"If doctors can learn meaningful information, I'm glad to take part. I'm one of 350 bypass patients being checked years after their operations." As the doctor holds the strip of graph paper with my wiggle lines on it, I ask her, "What does it say? That I'm as healthy as I look?"

"I don't have your pre-operation chart here to compare, but it appears you're either an athlete or you haven't retired yet."

"I wasn't an athlete, but I grew up on a farm pitching hay, lifting bales and manure until I was thirty. I walk three miles most mornings." Our banter is light and we tease each other. The doctor asks, "You're funny. Did the sense of humor arrive after the heart operation?"

"I always liked humor," and after a moment of thought, "but I think it has blossomed more since." JJL would have used other words other than blossomed to describe my humor: afflicted, pestilence or blighted would be her answer to that question.

I end up appreciating the young doctor's manner. "You looked me in the eye and listened to me as I answered your questions. How you relate to a patient is perhaps as healing as your medications," I inform her.

The ride home is easy and a delight. The trip is over and my heart appears to be OK.

I stop by to see JJL, and as I get a comb from her dresser, I make a discovery. "Guess what I found."

"My purse?" – She knows it right away! I'm surprised.

"Yes! I'll have to apologize to the ladies at the eye doctors, or you won't get your new glasses." I also breathe a sigh of relief. I don't know if she has credit cards or other things in the purse I would have had to call about. She doesn't shop, so I should take those cards. She says, "Nobody can get my driver's license." That is because the State cancelled it due to her mental instability. If someone drives with it now and is stopped, he or she could get fined for driving with an invalid license.

Self can't help getting my attention with, "I note she keeps her backseat-driving license current." He's a real scamp!

At home, Latte meets me at the door and an episode with another female begins. She would not let me hold her when we first adopted her, but she has gradually come to let me do it for several minutes now that her mistress is not around. I pick her up and put her on my shoulder like a baby. She is content and begins to purr, which bothers me. The reason it bothers me is because her head is beside my hearing aid and her amplifier is turned to broadcast level. It also sounds like her motor needs an overhaul. Then this lady cat, formerly known as Mrs. Lickey, demonstrates her love. That rough tongue going across the hearing aid sounds like sandpaper on a tin roof. We both enjoy petting for several minutes, but this time she enjoys it more than I do.

Then Mocha arrives and wants a shoulder. I believe the cats do get lonesome when I'm gone very long. They had JJL for twenty-four hours a day. They may not have adjusted to her leaving as well as I have but it appears they are now adjusting.

Yesterday Mocha sat by the studio window to watch the birds feed just outside. She would raise a paw as if she wanted to play with them. If I can coax some squirrels to eat peanuts in the yard, the cats should really enjoy watching the activity.

I'm noticing a real change in Latte. She meets me at the door when I arrive after the day, and comes to me, looks up and says, "Mrr." She then lets me pick her up and hold her without any effort to get down as in the past. This morning she arrived in the bathroom, and I put her on my lap and started petting her. Instead of jumping down after several strokes, she settled down and remained for four or five minutes. Is she having post-traumatic stress after the loss of her mistress? When JJL was here for a half-hour this week, the Latte did not wish to sit on her lap. We took it to be a means of punishing JJL for leaving the cat alone. Perhaps she will get over it. I will take greater pains to notice and love her. Today as I sit in the red chair, each cat is lying beside me on separate high-rise pieces of cat furniture, something Latte has not done in the past. Another first for her is coming across Jacquie's desk and over onto mine as I am typing. She appears to need attention again.

I've been busy, so that has helped me adjust to not having my JJL here. Yesterday at a wholesale warehouse, I realized how fortunate I am that she went to the Chateau so easily. I met the mother of a student I once had. Her mother is in the hospital, and is told not to go home with the daughter but to a rest home. The mother will not agree to this, and the daughter is overcome with caretaker stress. The mother with Alzheimer's Disease fell and broke a shoulder. I again count my blessings!

Today is Super Bowl Sunday. I am losing a few pounds now that I can plan only my own diets. The Superbowl will not bother me, as I will watch it with Jacquie. I am not to take any food to the rest home, so we will control the urges that cause pizza, beer, pretzels, cookies and potato chips to sell so well this weekend. We may have some trouble hearing the game. After dinner the Sue likes to turn on her electronic gadgets, take the microphone and sing. She does it because she enjoys singing and the volume in her room is rather high. This doesn't bother JJL, as she listens to TV with earphones, and her roommate is all but deaf. We only have one set of earphones, so today we will use the set's speakers. I have my fingers crossed. We enjoy the game with some difficulty.

I brought a different type of jigsaw puzzle for her this week. It is about thirty-four inches wide but only twelve inches high. She can see to do the work at the top of the puzzle, a problem for her now. This will be a part of Valentine's Day. I also find a box of sugarless chocolates. I'm so tired I go home early for some feline petting and sleep.

On a nice Sunday I take JJL down the Central Valley to see the greening hills. The almond trees are awakening and showing a hint of the blossom colors they will dress themselves with in a few days. We have pea soup at a restaurant famous for it. A week later I have planned to take her to see the almond groves in bloom but we decide to stay at our house instead and watch the Olympics. The cats are soon on her lap and all goes well.

Before I took her to the Chateau it dawned on us that we could be apart and yet together. That doesn't turn out to be completely true. She knows I can cook and care for the house but she's not sure about my care of the cats. She checks the cats' food and water bowls. "Don! Water." I empty the water bowl, knowing just adding to it is not good enough. As I turn on the faucet she continues, "No. Not tap water. Use the filtered faucet!" Same song and record, I realize.

I've heard this before but I act surprised, "For the cats?" I ask with one raised eyebrow and my mouth gaping as if I didn't know better.

"Yes. Always, and don't you forget it!" Her eyes are boring into mine. She feels very responsible, but her alert response to my set-up pleases me. Alertness is a good sign.

As I finished my walk this morning I realized I wanted a soak in the tub. While she may not be home, JJL can still give directions about my behavior. "Don't use the tub, Don. You might fall and I'd not be there to help." I determine how I can get help if I need it. I put my cell phone beside the tub and unlock the front door so the firemen don't have problems getting in if I must call them. I run the water knowing I've met my need for a soak and her need for my safety.

As I step out and start drying myself I know I'm doing better. The stress is not present and I am able to sleep without waking until morning. I feel as spry as a septuagenarian can feel, certainly much better than a few months ago when our problems began. In fact, I find I'm enjoying being an old man, much to my surprise.

Part Three
Now We Know

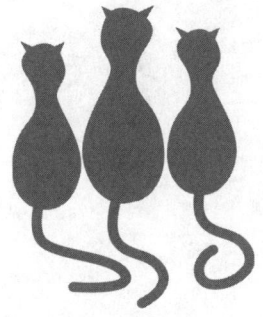

Chapter 29

Now We Know
Four Months Later

It's four months after JJL entered Chateau Livermore. Last night Larry called from Kansas and asked, "Hi Dad! How's Mom?" Since I have kept him informed of all the developments, I could keep the answer short. I wouldn't have to explain what we had found to be her problem.

"She's doing OK. She still has problems, but no more than she did the last few months. In a number of ways she's better than when you were here eight months ago."

It was late. The conversation did not last long. Larry was tired and upset about a fellow who earlier wouldn't accept help and enter his ambulance.

Larry had responded to a 911 call to go to a soccer field. The coach of a girl's team was feeling chest pain but refused to get into the ambulance. A team member's dad, a doctor, suggested strongly that the coach take advantage of ambulance. Just then a tornado siren sounded and everyone scattered. Including the coach. Larry's left with his ambulance empty.

"Are you OK, Dad?" Larry asked me asked before hanging up.

"I'm doing much better now that I am not stressed all the time. It's great knowing your mother is in good hands and is as happy as can be expected."

"That's great. I need to get the boys to bed, so I'll call next weekend. Bye now!" His medical experience helps him understand what is happening here with us.

Our short phone call quickly let him know how things are. Realtors at marketing meetings and neighbors ask, "How's your wife?" or, "How's Jacquie? And sometimes, "Did you ever find out what's wrong?" Answering the last question takes longer now that we know what the problem is.

"It appears she has dementia."

"How'd you find that out? A test or studying the symptoms?"

"Two weeks ago," I would explain, "I was ready to go to a marketing meeting when my cell phone rang."

I bought her a cell phone and programmed it for her ease of use. It is always on her walker within reach if she needs to call me. I don't call her, as she may be asleep or could become dizzy if she tries to reach it in a hurry. Having the phone is a comfort to her.

"The call was from Jacquie and she sounded frightened and weak," I tell my listener.

"Don," she said, "I wakened with both arms shaking and I couldn't stop them. Sue suggests it looks like Parkinson's disease to her. I'm scared."

"I'll skip the meeting and be right out," I assured her. When I arrive, I checked her pulse, blood sugar and blood pressure. All were normal. "I'll call the advice nurse," I announced as I reached for a phone.

"No. They will want me to come to the emergency room!"

I made the call anyhow. The advice nurse consulted a doctor, who wanted me to bring her to the ER, just as Jacquie had predicted, so we headed for the HMO facility. It was a long time before a doctor sees her, as there was a constant influx of ambulances with patients in a more serious condition. In time an EKG, blood serum test and a CT Scan were done. The nice tall Korean doctor said, "There is good and bad news. The bad news is that we don't know what the problem is, but the good news is that it's not coronary, stroke or other bad things we don't want to find." We were dismissed and came home.

"So you didn't find any problem?" people ask.

"Not then, but the trip did produce results. Ten days later she had a similar attack."

This time the advice nurse told us to report to Dr. Banda the next day. Everything checked out fine in her office. Then she pulled a green sheet from the file she received following the most recent ER visit. She read the report to us. It stated, "There is no subdural contusion or other evidence of head trauma." The second sentence added, "Diffuse generalized cerebral atrophy of a moderately advanced degree." Dr. Banda pulled out her pen and wrote, "Which causes Dementia," to finish the last line of the report. Evidently the CT scan was given a more thorough study later after we left the ER.

"Dementia," I say to my listener. "Her brain is deteriorating."

"Is there anything they can do for that?" my listener will then ask. Or the person will tell me of a friend or relative who is also suffering from dementia.

When Dr Banda wrote those three words her dark eyes looked into each of ours as and she asked, "You know about that, don't you?"

We both said, "Sure," and we left.

I learn later, I don't know much about dementia. It isn't that simple.

My sister and husband from the midwest come to spend a week with me. JJL is feeling better and spends two nights and three days with our company at home. That means watching and catching her as she starts to walk without remembering her walker. Using the walker is not a guarantee she won't fall either. It also means turning my depth of sleep control to one-third and my sense of awareness to high alert to sense if she gets up in the night to go for a drink or the bathroom without waking me. The last day of their visit, I return Jacquie to the Chateau. Then I take Phyllis and Owen to tour the USS Hornet, which is berthed in Alameda as a floating museum. An aircraft carrier has a lot of stories and many ladders to climb. After putting my guests on the plane I go home quite tired.

As I walk into the house, Latte, who heard the garage door, meets me. She walks beside me and stops when I stop. Looking up into my face she utters two small "Merrs," her new habit. I talk to her as I lift her to my arm and shoulder. She responds by purring in my ear and licking it with her rasp-like tongue. We walk the length of the house relating to each other in a loving manner. We need each other at times like this when Jacquie is not home with us. I am learning again the gratification of touch as it relates to love.

The next morning, "Self," I mumble, "We need to know more about dementia. Where can I find information in non-medical terms?"

Self replied quickly, "Try the Internet, dummy."

I do. I spend two hours reading and printing articles. There is a lot of very depressing bits of research. Few if any sentences or paragraphs are positive. Dementia appears to be a collective noun, like the word food, which covers many types of material from beverages to steaks to spinach. Dementia includes problems from Alzheimer's through a number of forms to an as yet unnamed version of the malady. One kind of dementia cannot be determined until the autopsy. Another Internet bit states only ten percent of the cases can show response to treatment. I'd better hold onto that as a hope. It is several days before I recover from my depression and tiredness.

Self reminds me, "You wanted to go the HMO medical library and do some more looking and reading." I go there this afternoon, and I am fortunate to be there at the same time as the library nurse.

"I will bring you some books and articles," she tells me. After hearing JJL is still falling this professional makes several suggestions I find to be quite good. "If she continues to fall," she says, "someone will have to make a decision how many falls a week is too many. At some point you may have to seek a home better equipped for this problem. As things become more difficult you will have other decisions to make."

"You mean a health plan like a business plan?" I ask.

"That's right. Your doctor can give you a lot of help along this line, as well as the rest home if you have a good one."

"I'll call Lori, the lady who helped us find this home," I announce. "I'll ask her if she also refers to homes at the next level up."

I call Lori the next day. "I specialize only in rest homes, Don," Lori tells me, "but I can refer you to a counterpart in the homes equipped to give more care." She goes on to give me background on the care of dementia patients and that helps. As we finish the call, she says, "I can tell you're more relaxed now than when you first called fifteen minutes ago." It is true. I'm feeling much better after learning more about how to deal with may be ahead. I'll think through what I've learned and begin to put together some planning on my walk to Safeway tomorrow. The quiet of a dawning day is a great time to think.

Mocha has heard me on the phone. Coming at a run, she jumps onto my desk and walks between the computer and me. Her tail dusts my face as she jumps to the roof of her apartment atop the scratching post. I've parked the post and apartment next to me to keep her from helping too much.

After the late news report, it is time to take my pills kept near the refrigerator before I go to bed. I am almost run over by Mocha, who dashes past me to stand by the refrigerator door. Looking up she gives me the "Here I am," sign. "I'm ready for my go-to-bed treat." She wins as usual. Next she will beat me to bed and wait for our go-to-bed petting. It is hard to remain uptight with such lovable diversions!

Latte comes onto the bed and the felines began giving each other facials while sitting on my legs and crotch. As usual, the facials end in a spat. Once a cat war erupts, you don't want them on your lap or crotch. I yelp and clap my hands. Each cat leaves the battlefield in one pounce and I once again relax.

I've been tired several nights. I'm tired quite often this month. Perhaps I'm stressed from my recent medical schooling. I don't feel like starting a project in the evening as I usually do. Since I've never been an old man before I might attribute this tiredness to aging, and then Self says, "Don, in the evening you should sit down in your recliner, after all you get up at four-thirty to start your day." I don't want to sit and do nothing but I need rest. I sit down and find a TV program. The next thing I realize, I am awakening to find it is after midnight. I'm not alone in this napping. There are usually one or two cats sleeping on my legs. Turning off the paid programming that appears after midnight, I take my last pills and fall into bed.

Mocha hops onto the bed and with her eyes on mine approaches to four or six inches of my head to see if I'm still awake. She flops down with her head in my armpit and her back against my ribs and begins to purr. I pet and manipulate the oversized pelt that fits so loosely around her little body. In a few moments she will get up and flop down on her other side. The petting and purring continue. It is then time for her to turn end-for-end and lie with her large hairy tail across my face. After five minutes she arises and hops off the bed to find another place to sleep. Latte comes to inspect my legs for a bed site. She prefers to sleep between them but if I am on my side she will lie beside my legs and curl into her fetal sleeping position.

I find myself starting to design the health plan. If I think about it seriously, I will not get to sleep. "Turn off your mind, Don, and go to sleep," my hidden partner commands. "I mean it now!"

Sleep arrives but it is a middle grade sleep and in a small package. I have an unhappy dream and I waken at two fifteen. The question arises, "Shall I take a sleeping pill or try to get back to sleep on my own? If the medication really works, I might miss the Realtors' marketing meeting. Oh, oh, worrying again. And besides, I took two pills last week. I don't want to become dependent on them. I did nap in the chair for several hours so maybe I'm not too far from my usual six hours of sleep". I do not sleep well. I know I will be yawning later in the day. The cats do not have a good night either as I kept turning and rolling in my troubled sleep.

Coming home from the meeting I try to visualize a Health Flow Chart in my mind. As an artist, I can see a new watercolor in my mind before I pick up a pencil or brush. This morning I have problems seeing a finished health chart. It will have to wait until I have paper and pencil. I do not have enough information to go beyond two or three levels of a chart.

The first level states the problem,	Dementia	
The second level box asks,	"treatable?"	
The third level has two boxes:	"If yes, how?"	"If no, Care not Cure — similar words but worlds apart in meaning
The fourth level asks,	"What's next?"	
	When _____	_____
	Drugs _____	_____
	Care _____	_____

Perhaps the beginning working chart isn't so bad. While I can't predict needs too far into the future, it gives me a sense of direction, and with the doctor's help it can be revised as time and conditions change. I do not put the chart into a finished form. I simply address a letter to

Dr. Banda listing the questions I have as I think about the chart and our future. I also add observations of both positive and negative signs my Jacquie is showing. I await a reply and will value her judgment.

I go to visit Jacquie as usual but she is depressed. She doesn't say why. She has a birthday this week. It must be depressing to think of celebrating her first birthday in a rest home and having to depend a lot on other people. I like to take her little gifts but that is difficult. When you share a room you don't have much space to store gifts. Flowers are welcome but she has allergies. She appreciates food but she is a diabetic I have to be careful of the sugar content of treats I bring; besides bringing food is against the sergeant's rules. I smuggled in a little square of gingerbread today and JJL is quite pleased with it. Maybe having it sneaked in past the sergeant makes it more attractive. My showing up with a big smile and a big, slow hug is a genuine gift. "To have and to hold, in sickness and in health," is easily repeated early in life, but I have found that both of us need, enjoy and treasure those moments of hugs and hand holding in each decade of our marriage. The looks in the others eyes are also a delight not to be missed.

Later at home I turn out the light and pull the bedclothes to my chin. In the darkened room, I can picture the smile on her face and the happiness in her eyes as I entered her room two hours ago. I smile to myself, remembering the happiness I felt at bringing her pleasure when she needed it most. I too had a warm, good feeling I shall not forget. I must keep myself strong as we are both depending upon me. I need to extend my health plan to include a box for me, find a support group locally or on the Web to maintain a positive attitude and strength.

I didn't know that such satisfaction is available in elderhood, but I've never been an old man before!

Chapter 30

The Weekend Date
She Is Home Again

I'm too tired to give her as much attention as she wants as I crawl into bed. I turn off the lamp and she snuggles closer to me. I fall asleep rubbing her neck and shoulders and stroking her back. "Why do you always want attention when I'm so tired?" I ask before I doze off. I don't know if she answers but she gives up and goes to sleep also. This morning I waken with pains in my shoulders and thinking of coffee and aspirins. She is at my side making sweet noises into my ear and asking again for my exclusive attention. She wants the caressing to begin again. I believe she thinks it should start at this moment. It's not hard to read her mind.

"I guess you want some loving," I say as I start to repeat the sequence of last night. She closes her eyes and displays a contented smile. She's winning. I'm still too tired and sleepy for much attention giving. Yet, as she is so demanding, I continue. In a few moments she turns and places her soft back against me. "She truly loves me," I say to myself. The caressing of her shoulders continues but only for a few moments. She turns while murmuring a line of my virtues but her fluffy tail tickles my nose. I sneeze a blessing to her. She's startled after the explosive sneeze. This young Birman cat lives up to the breed's characteristics. They are people lovers and are also known to be talkative.

I'm quite awake now. We both arise and stretch in the semi-darkness of my bedroom. Now that I'm awake, it looks like a good morning to sleep in. The late June fog of the San Francisco Bay Area is present with just a little wind caressing the tree tops, much as I caressed Mocha's silky back moments ago. Looking through the window, I see early ground-feeding birds feasting on the sunflower seeds I placed on the patio for them last night. There are a few peanuts in the fence feeder for the squirrels. I like to watch a scrub jay that isn't hungry place a peanut in his beak. He will hop to the fence to survey someone's yard as he prospects for a place to hide his booty. Watching this thief's energy makes my fatigue seem even more painful. "Aspirin, here I come," I say aloud to myself.

That inner voice I call Self, answers, "You can use that jay as a mentor, but don't expect to have as much energy as he displays. He's seventy-some years younger."

"Less energy or stamina is the downside of aging, Self. Today, I'll shave," I mumble. I've been forgetting to shave on Saturday mornings but remember it mid-afternoon. Forgetting was always an easy activity but now that I'm an old man I seem to major in forgetfulness. Perhaps I should consider starting a septuagenarian college. From a post office box I could sell framed degrees in Forgetfulness 101 for thirty dollars as a means of supplementing my Medicare. Wisdom 203 degrees could sell for more. The degrees would provide laughs as unusual gifts for hard-to-shop-for elders. It might be fun to go to retirement centers in Southern California and Florida on a sales trip or rent a booth at an AARP convention. All I need to do is to get Andy Rooney to mention it on his program.

"Enough of this foolishness even though it is your own time you're wasting," Self scolds me

"You're right. Today's to be a grand day. At my age, any day is grand, but I have a date. My wife, no less! I will get her after lunch and she'll spend the night at home with the cats and me."

This weekend's date is authorized and sanctioned by Sergeant Sue, Jacquie's little Philippine caregiver at Chateau Livermore, a residence converted to care for six ladies. "Sue, I would like to take my Jacquie for the weekend," I informed our new friend last night.

"You may have a date, "she retorts with her widest grin and eyes twinkling. She straightens up from her fit of laughter and raises a hand for a high-five. I slap her hand and she giggles again. "Just bring her back to me OK, hee, hee."

"What time is curfew?

"Seven o'clock. Prompt!"

"I'll see you tomorrow, Sue, when I pick up my date," I say with a nod of the head as I leave after my nightly visit with Jacquie.

"Be careful driving, Mr. Larsen," Sue shouts after me as always. Her military attribute of being in charge extends to me also. One more female is giving me directions. I learn a week ago how the Sergeant's standards can permeate the day. I arrive at five fifteen for a visit and Sue has JJL in bed. As I bend over for a hello kiss I note a sweet smell.

"You got powdered as you were dressed for bed," I state.

"You bet. We know now why Sue wants big cans of talcum powder." A month ago Jacquie told me about Sue's Powder Procedure 101. Imagine how I would smell if that big can of powder you brought was scented powder!"

"I've notice spots of powder on your couch, on the floor, in the closet and on the bath floor. I assume that's where you are dressed on different days. Right?"

"Yes!"

"I notice your new black wheelchair looks like a painter's truck. Instead of being splotched by paint and spackel, you have a nearly new black chair that is almost white. I think it is funny, Jacquie, but I also am glad she is caring. That's an important attribute." I have a doughnut with Dr. Grace, a ninety-six-year-old doctor, the next day and tell her about the powder regime. I inform this elderly medic, "After putting on an extra sweater on all her patients, the Sergeant opens all the doors and windows to air the house while the ladies are at breakfast." I end by saying, "Doctor Grace, the place smells fresh all the time."

"I'm glad," Dr. Grace states. "As a doctor I've gone to a lot of care homes and you could smell some a quarter of a mile away," she says with a twinkle in her knowing eyes and a smirk about her mouth.

Now that I'm shaved, I'll start the list of chores to finish before I bring Jacquie home. Planning to do a number of things seems to be easier than remembering to do them. "You are getting much more efficient at forgetting as you age," Self reminds me in a cocky manner. Starting my three-mile walk to the market and back as the sun rises gives me time to plan my morning sequence of events. Activating the sprinklers as soon as I arrive home will allow me to do some tidying in the kitchen and bedroom areas to avoid wifely suggestions on this home date.

Light classical music seems to hurry the clock this morning and it is soon time to stop the sprinklers, gather Mocha into my arms and to head for her eleven-thirty appointment with the veterinarian.

This longhaired white cat with lavender and tan blotches doesn't know about the appointment but takes things in stride. As a strictly inside cat, she notes strange odors as I put her cage into the car. As the car begins to move she murmurs low sounds of concern. We are on time but our doctor isn't. There have been several emergencies ahead of us, we're told. Now it's our turn and my feline has good behavior.

"Mr. Larsen," the vet states after the examination, "she'll be fine, but I want you to give her two quarter pills a day for two days and one a day for a week afterwards."

"How do I get her to take pills, Doc?"

"With one hand, pull her head back and after prying her mouth open put the pill into the mouth and push it down the throat with a finger."

"You've got to be kidding, Doc! A finger down the throat?"

"Down the throat!"

"Did you see that mouth full of teeth and how sharp they are?"

"Be quick, sir." With a smile he turns to leave, saying, "I've got another patient waiting for me." Mocha and I leave with a vial of pills. She's glad to be out of the clinic. I'm wrapped in thoughts of becoming a pill pusher. I don't put her into her traveling case but place her beside me on the seat. When we start moving she's soon on the car floor behind my heels.

As I pull out of the parking lot, the mouse on the computer screen of my mind deletes Mocha's appointment and moves to highlight JJL's icon and address. Rather than take my pet home, I'll take her to the Chateau as I collect my Jacquie. There's an interesting motive for this plan. I will take Mocha into the home filled with elder and handicapped ladies to let them pet her. It's easy to see how this cat brought life to their eyes on a similar visit a month ago. With the now calm cat on my arm I take her to the room of patients. The women straighten in their recliners and their eyes light up brightly. One comments, "How smooth and soft she is." Another who's lost in herself most of the time, awakens, peeks out from behind the blanket she keeps drawn over her face as Linus does in the Peanuts comic strip and asks as she reaches to pet Mocha, "What is it?"

The sergeant has JJL dressed and ready for our date with bags of medicine and clothes to accompany her. Jacquie takes Mocha from me and asks, "Mocha, did you come to visit me?" Petting and visiting with the cat is in order before I can guide my wife and her walker to the car. As I pull the front door closed I hear my latest orders, "Have a nice date. Drive carefully and bring her back to me Mr. Larsen!" As usual, a female, the sergeant, has the last word!

The weekend is going quite well. She is using her walker and I believe she is stronger. She is happy to be home and is enjoying herself. She doesn't overdo, as Latte finds her lap and JJL doesn't want to disturb the sleeping cat. As cats sleep a lot, JJL sits and I don't have to worry about her getting up and falling. I don't know it yet but future weekends will find a lot of sitting, as we will watch the final months of the baseball season. A few weeks after JJL goes to the rest home neighbors tell me, "Don, you are looking much better than you did before Jacquie went to the home." I notice she also looks better. I think she was worried about me.

I begin to look forward to our anniversary at the end of June. It will be fifty-five years this time. "What will you do this year?" Self, who has been monitoring my thoughts, asks in my right ear. "Go to the Claremont Hotel again?"

"I don't know as I haven't thought about it. She's better than she was a few months ago. I'll plan something." This will be something to think about on my morning walk Monday morning. The celebration won't have to be spectacular; rather I'll make it memorable in little meaningful ways. Bringing back memories and appreciating her progress since our disastrous fifty-fourth should be fine. Little do I know the day before the celebration will be more memorable than the anniversary itself.

Chapter 31

Can We Celebrate this One?
Fifty Five or Bust

It is a week later and another morning when it is sheer agony to awaken. The eyes can't eliminate their fuzziness, the elbows don't want to prop me up on the bed and the legs don't respond to my orders to move. Transforming myself from a happy sleeper to an alert being is a painful process. As I age I notice that this early morning transition becomes less fun. The old excitement of awaking and bouncing out of bed as in the past is missing.

I remember a conversation with a professor before a small biology class began at college more than a half century ago. "I love to take my time getting out of bed and I take even more time to dress," he declared.

"I can't do that," was my comment. "After waiting restaurant tables at night I go home to study into the night. But I did jump out of bed and into my clothes before sprinting to class." I thought this man was lazy or perhaps weird. There was never time to laze about on the farm where I grew up as a boy during the Second World War.

I wonder if the professor was going through what I'm experiencing now.

Putting memories aside, I am awake. It is four seventeen. It will take an aspirin and a cup of strong instant java to bring me up to speed. This will be a great weekend if I can pull it off correctly. In hours I will learn my JJL is having an interesting morning that in time might be remembered as quite funny.

I find it light enough to walk to Safeway and visit with the restocking crew as I do several times a week. However, I'm not feeling very energetic. "That first coffee must have been regular rather than high octane," Self smarts off.

"My body must need a tune-up. Hopefully it is to be our big day today." I know there is a lot to do before we can celebrate, if indeed we can. I'll not walk again until Monday, as I won't dare leave the house tomorrow morning with Jacquie home and subject to falling.

Back home, Self tries to give orders. "Don, if you're that bushed now, you need double-strength coffee. Drop another spoonful in." Reaching for the jar of crystals I can almost taste the stronger aromatic fluid.

After a shower, dressed only in underwear, I start to put water into what will be my second cup of instant coffee. I feel a wet rasping on my bare leg. Latte is telling me, "I always have cuts on any morning list of chores. Remember?" Experience has taught me that if licking doesn't produce the instant results she wants, she'll resort to nibbles on my leg. This thought causes me to set my cup down and do a barefoot dance as I get her moist cat food. Latte doesn't draw blood but her succinct message cannot be overlooked. Hearing the refrigerator door close and the spoon drawer slide open, she knows food is on the way and she goes to the feeding area. On mornings when I remember the tongue and nips as I arise, I wear trousers to the kitchen. On those days I'm able to have first dibs on the first treats of the day. Then, as my coffee heats, I feed her and Mocha, her feline roommate.

As I sip my morning wake-up fuel Self jumps into my mind to promote plans for the morning. "Don, first water the yard, get a haircut and phone about your defective new dishwasher. Also, a few other telephone calls need to be made. So get with it, now." He's been listening to JJL's mode of operation too much, I decide. I'd told Jacquie last night, "I'll pick you up in the middle of the afternoon." I check my watch. It will be several hours before those I need to call will awaken. The bank will not open early on a Saturday. So much to do!

I look around and see that Latte has walked off without eating. She wanted her food to be served, though she really wants to be able to eat it later. Females and their orders! Even though I'm ten or fifteen times her age, she demands priority and then flouts it in front of me. "Females!"

Watering the yard while enjoying my cup of instant joy is the first job on the list, on a quiet but delightful morning. The mockingbird is finishing his repertoire from a rooftop while the ground-feeding towhee chirps from the other side of the patio. The sounds and the smells in the pre-dawn air soon have me in the best of moods. I wish the essences of the pre-dawn air didn't leave with the darkness. I find the pureness of this time of day to be refreshing - a great tonic to both body and mind. I'm feeling well today. Cleaning the car's interior takes some time and also does not foul my attitude; however, there is a fouling of the air. There's the essence of skunk in our neighborhood. Some cat or dog must have surprised one that was late getting back to its den before dawn. I will become quite familiar with that odor in the next few weeks.

The car is finished, it is time to work on the house. Bringing JJL home for weekends means I always have a clean house for two days. She notices any spiderwebs I have missed or any of Mocha's white hair I have not picked off the carpet before she arrives. She makes these discoveries in the first few minutes of arrival. If the weekend is to be grand, it should start on the correct footing, everything in good order, no spiderwebs or Mocha's white hairs on the floor or recliners. I don't want to be a picked-on househusband! Becoming an older man often means a role reversal. Perhaps if the role reversal came earlier in life, we husbands might not gripe at our wives as easily as we did in the first few years of marriage. As an older man, I'm learning.

My morning chores are almost finished and the results are great. My satisfaction is heady and pleasing. "That's right, Don, a mirror would find you smiling."

"Thanks, Self, life is good for this old man today so far."

I've learned I need a break now and then for my own good. This is a hard lesson to learn. At break time I check a Wichita newspaper on the Internet for its obituary column. I can be aware of the passing of former neighbors and distant relatives. This interest developed as I became an aged member of society. I also keep up to date on other areas of interest. I find that wheat has reached three dollars a bushel. Self reminds me, "You remember when you sold wheat for four dollars in the mid-fifties?"

"Yes. I'm glad I left farming as a profession. No wonder the little mid-western towns have joined many Sierra communities as ghost towns!"

Back to reality. It is time to restart my chores. I shut off the computer before petting Mocha. She's sleeping on the flat roof of her condo atop the cats' scratching post beside my desk. She believes she is my assistant during my computer time. She reaches under my monitor and tries to catch the little arrow.

It's time to be off to run my other downtown errands. The list starts with a car wash and the removal of any white hair that clung to my trousers and now is stuck to the car cushion. Next is my haircut.

On my return, as I make a quick check of the house, I remember I've not told Sergeant Sue I want to take my wife for the weekend. I had better call the Chateau. "Sue, this is Mr. Larsen. I forgot to tell you I want to come out mid-afternoon to get Jacquie for the weekend."

"Oh yes," she giggles. "Jacquie told me you're going to get her every weekend." There are more giggles. I can visualize the twinkle in her eyes and the grin across her face. "She tell me you go to nice dinner. Good deal!" If her rapid and clipped speech is any indication, Sue enjoys our good times as much as we do. With four or five ladies to care for, she is unable to do outside activities herself, so she sees our activities as a highlight in her routine.

"Sue, today is our fifty-fifth anniversary. Tomorrow I'll take Jacquie to brunch at the Pleasanton Hotel if she is up to it."

"Oh yes, Jacquie she tells me" Sue giggles. "Have a happy anniversary!" I like this pleasant little Philippine lady. "I got her all ready for you now. Her clothes and medicine are all packed ready. She's waiting for you." Sue often mixes up her grammar, but her message is easy to read in her eyes and mouth. I look at the clock and it is only twelve. The Chateau's eleven o'clock lunch is barely over.

"I can't wait," I blurt, "I'm on my way to get her now. Thanks, Sue."

I learn upon arrival that it's a good thing I came early.

My wife is in the recliner designated for her in the home's living room. She is nicely dressed in a pink outfit and flashes me a warm smile. The smile quickly fades and she begins waving her hand in front of her face while she rolls her eyes in disgust. I've seen that sign for decades and I correctly guess the problem.

Poor JJL! I will have to rush her home and undo and redo Sue's thoughtful beauty shop type contributions and her idea of delights she lavished upon my wife. It isn't funny then but I know it will be a laugh in a few days, even for my suffering wife. Another situation I will not have had experienced had I not become an older, old man.

"I'll explain later in the car," she says. "I want aspirins as soon as I'm in the car. I hope my bottle of water is by my seat."

I put her into the car, shut her door and put her walker between the seats. Before I get behind the wheel she has opened the glove compartment to grab some aspirins I carry there. Then it's the bottled water.

"You smell rather strongly, very sweet and very pungent," I say. "That's the problem isn't it?"

"You'd better believe it." Her eyes are talking and her eyebrow sends signals as well.

"Sue was helping you? Did she spill it?"

"She had me dressed and I was sitting in my recliner when she came up and without asking rubbed some perfume behind each ear."

"Doesn't she know you are allergic to the stuff?"

"I thought so, but she was being kind and so pleased with herself. She did this final touch with a smile of pride. I think she is very happy for me."

"Will a bath as soon as we get home help?"

"I don't know but we'll try it. Sue didn't stop with the ear treatment; she came back and sprayed my hair with two shots of a different essence before I could tell her that was enough. She proudly told me she had bought the perfume at Macy's. It cost her ninety dollars for the bottle. She was very glad to share it with me."

"She did it because she wants to help you for our anniversary today and brunch tomorrow," I suggest.

"I'll never last that long this way. This allergy headache is killing me. Can't you drive faster?"

"I've never removed ninety-dollar perfume before." Another old man first.

Once in our garage she has her car door open before I can get to her side to help her. As I open the kitchen door for her, she reaches to activate the garage door closer switch, a tradition she's maintained over the years. Her brain may be atrophying, I think, but it is still quite sharp in a number of ways. Recently she is walking better, with less tottering. She may be walking on emotions only today. I have trouble catching her to steady her in case she loses her balance on the way to the shower. She's shedding clothes as we move through the house toward the bathroom.

"What'll it be? A shower or a drizzle?" I ask. We have learned to use a lawn chair and a shower nozzle on a hose for bathing. We call that new procedure drizzling instead of showering.

"A shower!" She reaches for a towel and I finish undressing her as the warm water flows from the showerhead.

"Stand here," I tell her as I shed my clothes, "so I can hold you to keep you from falling while you shower." In a moment we are soaping and scrubbing.

"I've got to wash my hair. She sprayed perfume on it, Don. Hold me now as I raise both hands to shampoo my hair."

In time the shower and redressing is over and the headache's on the wane. We spend the afternoon watching the Trans-bay baseball game between the Oakland As and the San Francisco Giants. Latte jumps onto JJL's lap, but soon jumps down. Jacquie spreads a lap robe across her legs with the green side up and the cat returns to make her bed and settle into sleep. This is satisfying to Jacquie. When Mocha alights beside Latte, my wife knows the feline facials they are giving each other will end in a spat. She is glad for the robe on her thighs, as it will protect her from claws when the disagreement starts.

It turns out to be a good day, and we will remember this fifty-fifth anniversary. Tomorrow we will have brunch if she is up to it. I've noticed she's better when there is a great need to be that way. We celebrate her good days and hope they last a long time before the dementia worsens. Earlier in the week Dr. Banda shrugged her shoulders and shook her head when Self prompted me to ask, "What is ahead for her and her dementia?"

I comment to JJL, "If tomorrow can be as good as today, we'll both have a great anniversary."

After the game she asks, "What's for supper, Don?"

"I don't know. The larder is empty. We'll go get something."

"No. We'll spend enough tomorrow."

"I have some stew but.."

I am interrupted as I expected. "Nope! Sue serves stew several times a week and I've had this week's quota."

"I have some popcorn."

"That's one thing we don't have because the other ladies don't have many teeth. Fix some." That sounds like an order from a female commanding officer. I have noticed how she is acting more forward than during the past few months, a good omen.

"Coming up."

"Do you remember what we had for dinner fifty-five years ago tonight?"

"No. Do you?"

"We rode with Uncle Carl to Wichita after the wedding. It was late and the restaurant in the hotel had closed, but someone brought each of us a sandwich."

"I don't remember that, but I remember we were the second wedding in your church that miserably hot and humid afternoon. We heard that Dennis, a high school classmate of mine, fainted in the June heat during his ceremony. Some of our guests' shirts stuck to the varnish of the church pews. Remember those little fans furnished to the churches by undertakers, with their name printed on the reverse side? They sure didn't do much air conditioning."

I hand my wife a bowl of popcorn. "It has butter on it," my spouse states with an upturned nose.

"It is butter-flavored. The package says it has fifty percent less fat."

"I don't care. Next time get the brand you used to get."

The eleven o'clock news ends and it is time for bed. After preparing us and putting her in bed, I lay back thinking about the day. It has been great. She is the Jacquie I knew. She had checked on me throughout the afternoon. She is in charge in her house, a good sign. Much of her memory is right on the dot, and she is alert to what is happening around her, whether at the home or around the world. She feels good, and when her balance is not a problem she walks well. In fact, she suggests we take walks on warm evenings when I visit her. We walk with her using me as a steadying force.

'You are holding up rather well also," Self reminds me. "Maybe the challenge she presents is a positive factor in your aging."

I respond, "I never guessed becoming an old man would be so challenging. I find it quite rewarding to be a bright spot in my handicapped JJL's life."

I take one last look at her sleeping and snoring on her pillow with Latte sleeping between her knees. I flash a smile heavenwards and fall asleep myself. Tomorrow could be interesting.

Chapter 32

I Talk Back To the Judge
Cat Husbandry With No Degree

"How was the art judging today?" my wife asks Friday evening.

"That's tomorrow," I answer her. Keeping dates and days correct is one of the problems dementia has dealt her.

I have looked forward to Saturday and it turns out to be quite a day, a day I will remember. I've judged county fair art shows for years but this one is unique. It is a challenge in several ways.

Fine art shows fall into several types: judged, juried or judged/juried. Often in places where there is little competition, the show is a judged show, meaning everything is displayed and the judge awards ribbons to only the best pieces. In places where there are usually more pieces submitted than can be displayed, the size of the show is controlled by a jury that selects the artworks to be shown and weeds out the less acceptable pieces – hence, the juried show. If ribbons are awarded after jurying, it becomes a judged/juried show. This is a judged show.

"Last year's show had problems, didn't it, Don?" Self asks as I near the fair site this Saturday morning.

"Yep! Even if there was only one painting to a class, we judges were told to award a first prize regardless of quality. As a result some poor paintings garnered awards while there were better paintings in larger classes that did not receive any recognition. It bothers me when the show superintendent insists on that."

When I arrive, I am met by an official named Charlie. "We changed the rules this year," he tells me. "We're going to use the

Danish system but also give awards."

"This may be a new twist," I whisper to Self. "Let's listen."

"You judges will give all the poor paintings a yellow ribbon, the middle quality ones are to receive a red ribbon and the best pieces are to get blue. Then the blues might or might not receive first, second or third place ribbons, depending on the opinions of you judges as to their quality."

"So a painting could get a blue designation but not a placing of first, second or third and money?"

"Yes. We'll make more changes next year."

"OK. I can do that. That's the way the youth art is handled in most fairs."

That judging change is not to be my problem. The first of several problems comes with the number of classes, or groups of paintings with similar subject matter. Examples of classes are portraits, people, domestic animals, wild animals, gardens, and flowers. This show has eleven classes in each of the six or seven media, such as oils, pastels and watercolors. This means there are probably seventy classes in the amateur division, and there is a duplicate set-up for the beyond-amateur group – in other words, way over a hundred categories to judge.

Self has been with me on enough judging to understand what's ahead and whispers, "Some deal you got yourself in this time, Don. I think I'll find a corner and catch up on missed sleep."

Charlie repeats his directions when the other two judges arrive. "Also, you'll need to choose the best for each media and then best of show for each of the two categories." We're glad the professional painters enter a separate show later in the year. We have enough for one day.

The next problem is to be one of my fellow judges. Sherry takes much more liberal posture than I am. "Don, I want you to stand your ground," Charlie tells me before the other two judges arrive. "One lady is rather strong willed." He's right, I am to find. It'd be easy to dismiss her as far out, yet she knows art principles and is a hard worker. She's thorough and consistent. I prepare to dig in when we differ. The third judge, Heddy, tends to vote with Sherry but she is not as vocal or dogmatic.

We start as individuals and do a lot of comparing and discussing; just what should happen in the judging process. If all judges agreed, then only one would be needed. We negotiate and make pointed comments about each other's tastes.

"Heddy and Don, I really like where this artist is trying to go. I say it should be a blue," Sherry says about a landscape where the bright green of the foreground doesn't grey with distance. The result is a "flat" painting with no definition of distance.

"Perhaps," I say, "but this guy signed George, didn't get where he was going! I'd give it a yellow. What do you think, Heddy?"

"I agree with both of you but I would go red."

That is the reason for a jury, to discuss and resolve differences. We each look at the painting again and more closely this time. I appreciate the ladies' desire to view each piece up close as well as from some distance. This means we take turns climbing a tall ladder to examine those works hung high.

While we all examine the craftsmanship and concepts of the works, Sherry is most concerned about, "What's the message the artist wanted to send?" Looking me in the eye, she continues, "Don, I know you're a realist, but this is great."

She is right, I am more interested in the visual aspects and beauty of the work. After telling her I had won top ribbons for my own abstracts, she tried to get to me when she saw an abstract she didn't like: "That's the kind of abstracts you paint?" We do agree on many pieces. We finish as strong judges respecting each other.

I left home at seven a.m. to make the long drive and arrived thirty minutes early so I had a chance to preview what was ahead of us. It is a tired old man who arrives home at eight p.m. Perhaps I am too old to tackle that sort of thing anymore. "You enjoy it, and you have several more fairs to go this summer," Self reminds me.

"Yeah, and I also believe such challenges keep me from aging as quickly as others." But this Saturday night I believe such days age me prematurely. I take aspirins and a hot soak before I go to bed early.

As I soak I'm glad I suggested to Charlie that he do as I did when I was art superintendent of our county fair show several years ago. "I eliminated all classes and media designations and told the judges to pick the best twenty paintings for prizes. We then divided the prize money twenty ways. Quality ruled rather than classes."

"We have to do something. The process we use has problems," was his reply. I understand the traditional process well. As an artist, I played the game of entering the classes and media groups that were weak in a show the year before. Of course when I became superintendent I had to stop entering that show.

It is not hard to get to sleep tonight. I usually think about many things before the sandman comes, but not tonight. Tomorrow I'll be tired, but it will be a restful day. I'll bring JJL home and we'll just sit watching a baseball game.

How wrong I am on that thought!

"Aspirins!" my shoulders scream upon awakening this Sunday morning. Before I can become too worried about my aches I have the comfort of knowing someone cares about me. Mocha notices my awakening and is within inches of my face checking that I really am awake. "You're my little sweetheart," I say as I stroke her body. We lie in bed purring and scratching before it is time to start the day on my feet. How could I know she would be a major problem to me later in the day?

While doctoring my mug with an extra measure of caffeine crystals I wish I had someone to rub liniment on the part of the back I can't reach. Eating my corn flakes I think of the females I will soon meet when I go to the Chateau for JJL. I picked up an antenna doll for Sergeant Sue's doll collection.

I will try to make up for not being able to see JJL yesterday, the first day in the six months she has been at the Chateau that I have not been there. Yesterday afternoon she called me on the cellular. When I answered she exclaimed, "I'm glad to know you're home already."

"I'm not home, I'm still at the fair. We have another twenty paintings to judge, and then we need to pick the Best of Show painting. I won't see you tonight, as I can't be there before closing. I'll bring you home tomorrow."

"I've got things to tell you, but I'll hang up so you can get back to judging."

The aspirin and the coffee are helping this morning. I sit with my feet in our conversation pit while I put on my shoes with the snoopervising help of Latte. She is becoming quite friendly with me now that her mistress is not around the house most of the week. This feline queen comes to me and verbally asks for petting rather than slinking off as she did in the past. Today she seems to be saying, "You were gone all day yesterday and it looks like you're leaving again."

"I'll soon be back with your mistress. She'll spend the day with us."

An hour later Sue opens the Chateau's door. "Happy Sunday, Mr.

Larsen. You come for your Jackie? She ready for you!" This short little lady is standing as tall as she can and grinning as usual.

I reach out my hand with the Jack-in-the Box antenna ornament concealed in my fingers. Here is a tiny doll for your collection."

She jumps several hops backward. "What is it? What is it?" she asks in a high, frightened voice. "No. No." I reveal Jack and then the big black eyes smile as she takes the gift. "Thank you. Thank you very much, Mr. Larsen."

It doesn't take long to change Jacquie from house slippers to sandals, and soon we are on our way home and a quiet day of resting. It's true; it is restful for awhile. "What was it you wanted to tell me yesterday when we were on the phone?" I ask. "Something I need to get for you?"

"No. I was going to tell you how I goofed at the table. You remember Nel, the one who won't eat?"

"She's the one who takes food from her mouth and puts it back onto the plate when Sue looks the other way, isn't she?"

"She's the one. Maribec, the Chateau owner, visited the other day and brought cupcakes. She arrived as we were sitting down to eat. Nell, who never talks to anyone, saw the treats and straightening up she asked, 'Can I have a cupcake?' 'You have to eat most of you lunch first,' Sue stated as she put a spoonful of lunch in Neil's open mouth. 'Now can I have a cupcake?' Nell asked. 'More bites first.' The lady is a con artist. Did I tell you about how funny it was after she had made a mess during the night? After Sue had her changed and clean it was time for a diarrhea pill. Sue put the pill into Nel's mouth and she took a swallow of water. To be sure things were right; Sue had Nell open her mouth. The pill was gone. After Sue left the room, Nel reached up and retrieved the pill and threw it under the table."

"But what happened yesterday you wanted to tell me about?"

"Nel was being obstinate again at breakfast and I whispered to the lady beside me that Sue should have some cookies so Nel would eat. I whispered too loud and Neil's sharp ears heard me. 'Cookies! Can I have a cookie?' she asked loudly several times. I should have known better."

"I'll bet Sue sent you an very clear message via her facial language."

"She did!" Then Jacquie changes the subject, "Let me help you with the lunch." It is not a question; the tone is declaratory.

"I don't have much to fix. Remember, I got home late and tired last night."

"We'll find something. Let me see what you have." So, holding her arm, I guide her to the kitchen. "Oh, you have two roasting ears. Sue doesn't fix them for us as most of the ladies have bad teeth or no teeth at all. We've got enough here, so let's not go out."

We have lunch ready before the Giants game starts.

After we eat, I take our empty plates to the kitchen and announce, "I'm going to the bathroom."

"OK." I find it interesting that now she's older she feels she needs to give permission to many of my actions. On the way through the bedroom I notice I have a problem. Mocha has been sick again. Like she did a month ago, the accident was on the bed. I put the comforter in the washer and then I return to the game. "You stayed in the bathroom long enough," I am informed. I think there is more scrutiny of my behavior than decades ago but on the other hand, I may be getting more sensitive or need more managing. I won't duck getting older because of these remarks. They're like fleas or flies. They're often present.

At the end of the second inning Latte goes to her scratching post and lies on her side, asking me to play with her. I poke a hand around the post for her to slap playfully. I remark to JJL, "My hands tell me it is time to trim this cat's nails.

Then Jacquie asks, "Where's Mocha? Is the little darling OK?" I go to check on Mocha. She must be ashamed and not feeling well, for she is in hiding. I can't find her.

At the seventh inning stretch I am informed, "You can probably put the comforter in the dryer and the sheets into the washer." Jacquie is right. As she takes naps in the afternoon and I am still quite tired, we nap through an inning and a half of the game.

Later, I make the bed. Jacquie and I go out for crepes at a pancake house and then I take her back to the Chateau. It's been a great afternoon but my weekend is not over. I do some homework and after the eleven o'clock news begins I head for the bed. Self says, "There's that smell again. Turn on the light."

"Oh no! Mocha, you've been sick again and at the same place." So at eleven- thirty I start the laundry process again. I read part of a book and only put two sheets on the bed before I crawl in. I begin thinking about a presentation I will make Thursday to a group of Realtors. I don't think about it long as I am soon asleep.

In the morning I start to awaken casually but something is wrong. "Oh no, not again!" I have towels on the pillows for the cats to sleep on so they won't get hair on the bedclothes, but one towel did not extend down far enough. Then I remember in a fit of half sleep hearing a cat pawing the bed covers. Since Mocha plays on the bed for fun, I did not come full awake. I am now wide awake and stripping the bed for the third time in twenty-four hours. She'll go to the vet for sure today, I vow. Last night I had draped the almost dry comforter over the red chair and the cat's apartment on the top of their scratching post. Without thinking, I had created a covered retreat, and that's where Mocha is recuperating. We make a three PM appointment with Dr. Bird.

I am tired. I had a weekend like two or three rough days in the middle of the week. But I venture out. Today I need to deliver some reports and my marketing newsletter to a dozen real estate offices. "How are you doing, Mr. Larsen?" the receptionists ask.

"Not so good!"

"What's wrong?"

"I can't get started. I'm slow and tired. I try to shift into a faster gear and I think I must have stripped my gearbox. I'll have to get an extra shot of caffeine in a cup of coffee soon or I might not get home." I find the strong coffee does help but I cut the marketing short today.

I sometimes feel guilty with Jacquie in a care home. That worry may cause some stress resulting in a stronger blood pressure prescription for me. The eleven o'clock news this evening doesn't help me either. There is a report about a couple in San Francisco. He is in his eighties and has dementia. After treatment in a hospital he is sent to a rest home instead of to his home. His little wife is having a fit because he isn't home where she can care for him. "I've done it for fifty-two years. I know him. He will be happier." A TV reporter questioning the man finds he is not able to answer questions correctly. He fell in the rest home, and two of the care people weren't able to help him up so they called 911. But the eighty-five- year- old wife insists, "I can help him up if he falls. I've cared for him for fifty-two years. Let me take him home." The city has an ordinance about proper care of people and the case will go for a hearing before a judge.

I didn't anticipate that a situation would happen in a day or two where I might not be able to call 911. That's a frightening story.

Chapter 33

Fainting/Slipping In The Shower
I Can't Call 911

It is Sunday night three weeks later. I am tired but as I lie back on my bed there is a smile on my face. It has been a great weekend in spite of the emergency I experienced at the most inopportune time I can imagine. Fortunately, we survived the situation but it will be in my memory every time I shower.

Before leaving the Chateau Friday evening, I told Jacquie I would pick her up mid-afternoon Saturday. Early morning yard work went well, so I change my mind about the time when I'll get her. She enjoyed the sandwich I made for her on Independence Day, saying, "It's much better than we get at the Chateau. The food is nutritional there, but it doesn't taste like what you fix at home." Why not get her early and make her another sandwich, I ask myself.

"If the taste of the food is the only complaint you have against a care home, that means the cleanliness and care are satisfactory, in my opinion," I counsel her. "Friends tell me other homes aren't much to brag about in any manner."

"Since JJL's noon meal is at eleven, you had better drop your pruning shears and get ready to get her," Self reminds me.

I'll call Sergeant Sue to say I will be there before lunch. I'll pick up a quart of milk for JJL on my way to the home.

On the fourth ring of the phone I am almost ready for Sue's staccato answer, "GoodMorningChateauLivermore,thisisSue.Howmay Ihelpyou?"

"Slow down, Sue. You talk faster than I can listen.'" My ears have slowed over the years but I would welcome sponsoring Sue in any fast talking contest. Her speech generator has a very fast microchip and an equally fast speech PA system.

"OhHelloMr.Larsen. Hee, hee, hee. You come to get your Jacquie, yes? She wonders what time you come for her. I gotherready."

"I didn't see you when I left last night to tell you I would get her early," I fibbed. "I'll give her lunch at home."

"OK. She like that. She ready now for you. She's looking for you. Hee, hee. I got her clothes and medicine all ready now."

"I'll be out within the hour. I'll bring her back in time for bed tomorrow night. OK?"

"That's OK. She likes that. She ready to go! Be careful now." Sue has a protection overlay or safety default built into her thinking or at least her talking. She has some warning advice for me each time I see her. That is good in her line of business. I do appreciate her motherliness to Jacquie and towards me also. She is a caring person who likes her work and is not doing it just as a job. In decades past we used to call that type of caring as dedication. People looked out for each other in the small communities whether related or not.

Clean up the kitchen before you leave to get her, I counsel myself. She'll check orderliness as she comes into the house unless Latte hears us arrive and is waiting by the door. If Latte is there she will be distracted from checking my housekeeping. I could have skipped the cleaning as Latte meets us. Jacquie bends over to greet her and the kitchen orderliness is missed.

"Hello Latte. How's my kitty?" As JJL pets the cat, she receives appreciative licks on her hand from this dark Siamese. "Where's Mocha?" Jacquie asks. The cats have become a very important part of her life and perhaps the cheapest medical factor in Jacquie's well being.

There will be other cheap entertainment to give her happiness today. I did the planning on my pre-dawn walk yesterday. There will be an afternoon ballgame and we will sit beside each other while Latte sleeps on JJL's lap. I have several lamb chops in the refrigerator. Jacquie has enjoyed lamb ever since we had raised them on the farm a half-century ago. She doesn't get lamb at the Chateau. As she appeared strong and stable when I saw her Friday I think with help she might like to fix the dinner. When the game ends I fib, "I have some lamb chops, but I'm not sure how to cook them. Would you like to come to the kitchen and advise me? I'll get you a chair."

"Yes. I saw the lamb in the refrigerator. Forget the chair."

I have to get up and follow her with a hand on her arm in case balance becomes a problem. She doesn't stop for her walker. Things are looking up.

While she watches the chops on the grill I wonder aloud, "Would you like a roasting ear and some canned beans?"

"Yes to both." Cooking in her own kitchen and directing me to do what I already knew seems to bring back her self-confidence. Later, we will watch the news at six and see mid teen girls taking several days of fire fighting training. They will not become firepersons, but this activity is to gain confidence in themselves. In my JJL the cooking is for the same purpose and perhaps as good as several of her pills.

Not knowing what is next in the script for her disease or any way of predicting it, I plan to make each day a good one for her. "Is it OK if I come out to see you each day, Jacquie?" I asked six months ago when she went out the Chateau.

"You'd better if you know what's good for you," was her answer. Her life and health will worsen, but when and how is yet to be learned. Dementia is a collective noun, as is the word color. Color takes in everything from black to white and differs when one shifts from pigment colors to the colors of light. Science has explored and examined the world of light, but we only at the beginning of dementia discoveries. Alzheimers is a dramatic variety of dementia, and one we hear a lot about, but there are many other forms. Presently, one type of dementia can only be determined at the time of an autopsy.

Coming home from visiting JJL last weekend I turned on the news. "An eighty-year-old-lady in San Ramon," a town ten miles north, "with Alzheimers walked away from a grocery store while shopping with her son. She is dressed in white. Anyone seeing her is to call…" I hoped for the next several miles that my Jacquie would have a less severe form of this malady.

As we go to bed Saturday night Jacquie asks, "Don, be sure to wake me in time for the Sunday Morning program with Charles Osgood. You'll be up before I waken."

"Can't you watch it at the Chateau?" I respond.

"We had it going last Sunday as we were all sitting in our recliners in the family room while our beds were being made. Then the other ladies asked Sue to get some cartoons. I missed most of the program."

"OK. I might also have breakfast in bed for you, good night, sleep well." If her ego and her need to feel needed can be stroked, having breakfast in bed should be on target.

In the morning I bring her a tray loaded with muffins spread with fruit yogurt, milk and a half banana. I have to remember her diabetes meal-chart serving sizes. "Don't forget the pills and insulin shot Susie packed for me, Don." The pills and insulin are also served in bed as the TV program comes on. She has company, as I sit on my side of the bed and the two cats stretch out on the towels I have on the pillows tops.

"At the Chateau I usually take a short nap after breakfast so I'll stay in bed. If I doze off, don't let me sleep too long because I want to take a shower."

I position the old red rocker in the living room so I could see her in case she starts getting up without her walker. I am tired and want to relax. Last, I turned my mental sleep control setting to, sleep light, last night so I'm more aware of her movements and I'm not fully rested.

The next thing I know is her hand on my shoulder. "You went to sleep." She has her walker, thank goodness. "Let's shower now. OK?" I don't expect the crisis what would occur in the next few minutes.

On the way to the bathroom she notices that there is only a little water in the cats' water pan. "Get water for the cats, Don. I'll hold onto the chair." I start to fill the pan and she issues a change order, "No. Don't just fill it. Empty it and put fresh water in it." I started to follow orders and then have yet another change order. "Not water from the faucet, use the filtered water we use for drinking."

"She's said that before! She's not doin' bad this morning," Self notices.

I help her to the bathroom. As I turn on the water, she takes two towels. "Can't Jane get the towels on the right shelves?"

"When she comes every other Friday, what she finds is dirty towels. She doesn't know where they came from, Jacquie."

"She has some kitchen towels mixed with bathroom towels." JJL's pretty sharp as Self implies, I say to myself.

"The water is ready. I'll undress you and help you into the rear of the shower."

"OK Don, but you shower first and then hold me."

"It won't take but a minute to get the plastic chair and install the hose with the nozzle."

"No. You just hold me like you did before two weeks ago before you got those things."

I shower while she holds onto a grab bar that I installed a year ago. Still soapy, I step behind her and hand her the soap. Soon she is soapy, too. How can I hold her safely? She had two protrusions on her chest but both they and my hands were quite soapy. They would not be a safe or substantial hold anyhow. I interlock my fingers from both hands just under her breasts. I soon realize it is a good thing I took this precaution.

"Don, I'm getting sick." Her head drops forward and I feel her body go lax. I grip my fingers tighter and steady my legs against any eventuality. "I'm getting weak, hold me," and she starts to slump. "You gave me my insulin shot didn't you?"

"Yes. Jacquie, can you turn to the right to get a hold on the grab bar?"

"Nnnoo," is the sound reaching my ears. She's out.

`I wonder if I can hold her, let alone help her.

"If you try to let her down by squatting," Self says, "you're liable to slip on the soapy water and have another problem even if you don't break the glass doors."

I reply, "I can't yell loud enough for neighbors to hear. We insulated the house quite well when we built it. Besides the two closest neighbors are gone. Her soapiness will not let me let her slide gradually to the floor. It will be all at once and crash. If I had my cell phone, but I don't have a pocket for it dressed this way. No 911 cellular call can be made at the moment. I can see Latte through the shower door but she can't help."

What if I could reach 911, I asked myself. The front door is locked and bolted. I would have to tell them to kick in the door at the back of the garage and come into the house there. I can't hold her long enough for them to get here. I will have to get her down so blood can reach her head to help revive her. If I slip and she falls onto me we will make a pretty sight for the firemen. If I knock myself out on the tile walls on the way down, I'll not see the firemen perhaps. Tonight a fireman's child might ask, "Daddy, did you have any interesting rescues with your fire truck today?"

"No. We just had to rescue a lady who fainted in her house," he'll answer with a wink at his wife.

There is a slight movement in Jacquie's body as she begins to come back to me. In a minute or two more I ask, "Can you turn with help and hold onto the bar?"

"I think I'm coming back. I'll try."

"Hallelujah. I don't like the alternatives if you don't." In a moment she is able to turn. I hold her with only one arm as I pull a towel from the shower frame and begin to dry her. She leaves the shower with more moisture on her body than ever before, but she is soon in bed and coming back to reality.

"It seems to be my stomach. I thought I would lose my breakfast."

"I'll get dressed, and when you're up to it I'll dress you. Meanwhile, rest."

She is soon asleep, as has been her mid-morning habit for a year. Soon Latte jumps onto the bed, finds a comfortable spot on JJL's thighs and joins her mistress by napping also. Mocha has chosen my pillow for her cot.

An hour later Jacquie wakens to find the Sunday papers on the bed with the comics spread out for her. When she finishes the paper it is, "Don, help me get dressed as I need something for lunch."

"A light lunch perhaps?"

"Yes. What time does the Giants game come on? If it's on now, tune to it." She is back with me. After dressing, lunch is served and we enjoy it. Later, I am asked, "Don, do you know you got several innings of a nap during the game?"

It is time for an evening snack and medicine for both of us. It is then that we go to what she calls her new home. "I have my home and Don has his home," she tells people. As I undress her and put her into her bed at the home she remarks, "I'm tired. Thank you for a nice weekend."

"I'm tired also," I say. "I apologize for forgetting to dump a handful of powder into the front and back of your nightgown as Sue would have done." My JJL wrinkles up her nose and sticks her tongue out at me. On the way back from the Chateau without her, I tell Self "I don't remember dates of fifty or more years ago as being quite so tiring, or more full of feeling and love."

It has been a good weekend. Her interest in the cats, home, me, a ballgame and a change of food are a great tonic for both of us. I benefited with a slower pace, having my wife home and seeing her so happy.

Chapter 34

The Day of the Female
A Miniature Prim Lady

I am leaving the world of sleep and its comforts. As I turn in bed to check the time I feel a light tread on my bed. As my eyes struggle into focus I see it is Mocha checking on me. As she approaches to within four or five inches of my face to see if I am awake, I tell her, "Mocha, it is too early, and there's no moon for my walk."

"Mrrr, mrrr," she purrs as she flops down beside me. She begins to massage my ribs with her front paws, probably as she did as a kitten nursing her mother. I stroke her long silky pelt, I can see her eyes are closed and she has a smile on her face. Her purring is almost too soft to hear but I can feel it as I pet her. It is as if an off-centered flywheel is revolving to vibrate her small body. She flops onto her other side and turns end for end several times before ending her morning greeting session.

"Oh no," I cry aloud as I see her move towards Latte who is sleeping a few feet away on another part of the bedspread. There will be female wrestling on my bed this morning. This is to be the first performances of many today. I sprint to the kitchen to start my coffee and it is time to cry, "Oh no," again as Latte rushes to the kitchen also. I hadn't stepped into trousers so I knew she would be communicating both her love of me and her message of, "I need food now before you get java." Her communication is delivered with her sandpapery tongue on my bare leg, which is bad enough. If she becomes disgusted with my non-instant service she resorts to nipping the unprotected calf. She has me trained to drop everything and move her to the top of the action list. She even gives me silent consideration by looking up and uttering a very soft meow as part of her promotional routine. It's the same as yesterday. I should learn.

Now dancing barefooted on my kitchen floor I feed her. "You darn females," I tell her as I stick out my tongue in her direction, "You made me wait for my coffee. I hate you!" Worse yet, she smells the food I set before her and tries to cover it by reaching out with her right paw and doing a covering motion before walking away. She isn't hungry but she wants it to be ready later. "Females!" She is number two today.

With coffee in the tasting mode I sit down with my coffee to watch the pre-dawn news. Guess what? It's a lady newsperson. She is good with diction, pace and eye contact. Her male team member has the day off. The day of the female is beginning. I wonder if Martha Stewart will be next.

I finish the coffee and pet the feline females one last time. Then I don my white cloth walking hat and step into the dawning day and some strictly male thoughts. Wrong! I see my neighbor Martha, mother of ten grown children, throwing bundles of the daily newspapers into her pickup for delivery. I also see the two young ladies I admire for their dedication to rapid walking turning right onto Colgate at the top of the hill. They walk with arms bent and swinging to match their pace and rapid conversation. They act like teens but they are probably in their thirties. I haven't seen them for several weeks so I turn and start around the block in the opposite direction so I can wave or say, "Morning," to them. I hardly get started at my old man default pace when they meet me.

With a grin the shorter one smiles and asks, "Do you see the smoke behind us?" I nod, and think, more females, but like our cats, I appreciate these ladies. The next female will surprise and challenge me in a few minutes.

I pass through the side yard of a friend's vacant house and enter a field of several acres. As I watch where I step to avoid turning my ankle on the plowed ground my peripheral vision makes me aware of some movement to my left. Sure enough! It is big and black with its large black tail quite erect. Its long tail bristles stick out at right angles from the tailbone proper like a black bottlebrush. A snowy V starts between the ears and tapers back over the hips. The contrast between the white stripes and the black fur is beautiful. The intent of this skunk is not as beautiful. Its eyes are on mine and its back is humped. With tiny front feet together it is making small jumps in my direction. As a midwest farm boy a half-century ago, I became acquainted with skunks. I detour around this animal and continue. On the way home, I walk near the same area. I find I had been near a burrow and wonder if this skunk was a female and returning to her kitts at home. I was a threat. There are many little digs where she has been digging a few inches for insects. This female doesn't make it home before the dawn is crowding out the moonlight.

As I walk by the shopping center, I note the only person outside of Lowes is a female watering the plants for sale. At Safeway most of the restockers working through the hours before dawn are also ladies. Now that I'm a bachelor, I do enjoy some conversation, so the quick comments with these familiar people fill one of my companionship needs. I choose several bananas and head home. As I wait for a cement truck to pass at a crosswalk in the now lightening morning, I note the driver is a rather small and pretty woman.

I finish my walk and call Donna, my daughter-in-law, to see if there are house inspection reports for me to deliver to Realtors, who probably will be female. No big deal, but I wonder where all the males in California can be.

Chapter 35

Thoughts And Rethoughts
I Get Away With It

I did it. I did it. I get away with it. And I should, I'm an old man and it's about time I started thinking instead of reacting by habit. On second thought, habit doesn't have a chance this morning.

Wakening at three-thirty, I can't get back to sleep. My brain refreshes at a quicker pace than my body. Mocha hops onto the bed to check on me and receive her customary petting for being a good watch cat. After thirty minutes the default sleep mode doesn't function so I decide to plan my day. I want to check my feelings about aging. That should not be hard as I have a lot of notes to draw upon. The problem is to write my thoughts in an interesting manner. Art Linkletter at ninety said he was over the hill but that is better than being under it. Telling a story is not as interesting as using conversation. Since I'm living alone, I don't talk to many people about my inner thoughts except Self. At least I can understand him. I comment on many things to the cats but I also visit with Self a lot.

Around five I notice that it is beginning to grow light outside. I say to Self, "I've decided to go for my walk after some coffee. I want to be back before the sun is in my face, so I'll put on my walking shorts and leave now."

"You mean you will go after feeding the cats. They'll get to you as you fix your coffee."

"Nope, I'll fox them." I will outsmart the felines. I will go directly outside instead of to the kitchen. There will be no licking or nipping my exposed legs to remind me to do feline feeding.

This Monday morning is a great one to start a week. Before I am five steps into my journey, I have taken two deep breaths of the unusually cool and humid air, a unique pleasure in a California summer. There is a high overcast and no wind. The promise of a nice walk is leading me up Lincoln Avenue. By the time I turn onto Colgate I notice something is missing. "What is missing?" I ask Self, who's always listening.

"Wha'da ya mean? What's missing?"

"There are no morning sounds."

"Such as?"

"There's no bird sounds. The mockingbird must have taken a break for a moment. Perhaps it is an entertainer's union break, although a lot of people don't consider night-singing mockingbirds to be entertainers. They describe these vocal fellows in more demeaning terms. There are no crows flying to the day's foraging areas. At this time on most Mondays the garbage trucks are making their distinctive noises. The only sound I hear is the Altamont Express slowing for commuters at the downtown stop."

"That train starts its run from Stockton, forty miles away, Self says. Those riders must have arisen before you did Don, to dress and board the train an hour ago."

"That's right, Self. Hey, it's still dark enough to see car lights coming into our valley over its four northern and eastern passes.'

"Watch it, Don! Stop a moment and you'll be OK I think." I had been looking at the stream of lights coming over the Altamont Pass and hadn't seen the immature skunk posturing in my path ahead. I waited a moment and it turned and hurried into the shrubbery.

"Oh look, a truck slipped into town during the night. It is backed into Lowe's unloading dock to await the store's crew to arrive at six and unload it."

"Don, you're right. I can see the driver napping while his huge diesel engine is resting with deep rattling breathing."

"Maybe it's snoring. Did you think of that?"

The Safeway restocking crew is busy as I arrive and I pick my way around the pallets of butter, yogurt and cheese. I don't know when acquaintances become friends but I am getting much closer to these people. They ask, "How is your wife?" without knowing my name.

And in return I ask several workers, "How much longer did you say it is until your retirement?" Or "How come cauliflower is so high? Are they using gold to fertilize it?"

Last Saturday, as I brought JJL home I stopped at the store with her. This time she was willing to come into the store to choose some things she would like that are missing on the Chateau's limited menu. Self whispered into my ear, "Don, she hasn't been willing to come into a store with you in months. She's changing for the better."

"Yeah, I notice," I whisper back. "I do think she is gaining more confidence in herself, I don't know why."

"I don't know either," Self confides, "but asking her what she wants said several things. First, you trust her judgement and you also want to please her. I think that helps her a lot. Too often folks placed in homes are forgotten or not given chances or choices." He's is right on target this time I believe.

Several employees in the store move to us to say hello to her and wish her well. Perhaps they are now qualified as her acquaintances. As I walk home this morning I smile to myself as I realize how much these people mean to me as I drift further from my former social scene, the scene of several years ago.

Self is reading my thoughts as usual and says, "I agree."

"I am no longer in contact with the school society I had prior to retirement. Time for care giving and helping our inspection business means cutting watercolors from my schedule. In turn, I cut night art association meetings and the traveling to enter and retrieve paintings from shows. Not doing inspections now means I can drop house inspection association meetings also.

"Yes," my inner companion notes and continues, "Meeting the clerks and stockers at the grocery as well as the Realtors and their office clerks as you distribute the inspection newsletters you write for the company has developed a new social network for you."

"This is what Jimmy Carter, ex-president, meant in his book, *The Virtues of Aging*."

"Yeah, I know, I read the book over your shoulder," my nosy partner informs me.

The book is small and can be summarized easily. "Upon retiring, expand all aspects of yourself - social, mental and physical - and your health will remain better than what doctors and pills can do to bring it back."

Back to the morning walk. Life is breaking out as I return to my neighborhood. "Oh look, Self. The crows are now commuting to feeding areas. The mockingbird has started his morning wake-up program as he stands upon a tall power pole." My eyes shift to the pair of fast-walking ladies almost running up Harding Street.

Noticing my turned head, my companion informs me, "Don, they walk too fast. You'll have to forget greeting them this morning."

"OK, but maybe I can bring Rosie to life in a few minutes when she comes out to get her paper." I walk by her house and put a banana inside the morning paper she will soon retrieve. Both she and I enjoy this silent communication. Perhaps this fits into Carter's philosophy.

Turning down my street I notice something flying at a rapid pace just above the housetops. "What kind of a hawk is that?" Self blurts out.

"It appears to be too big for a Kestrel." I turn for a second look.

As it comes out from behind a house and shoots upward in a rapid climb, my inner companion notes, "Look at those two doves headed away from the area for safety!" The hawk, hunting for breakfast wheels in a quarter circle, then dives at a tree I can't see, only to shoot into the sky again. It repeats this maneuver six or eight times before giving up and landing on a power pole. It is a Kestrel, often called a sparrow hawk. A pigeon takes flight from a nearby palm tree, while a small bird in the same tree remains on a frond ready to dash back into cover should the hunter change its target area.

Entering the house I win a second time over the cats. I read yesterday that though cats nap, their ears never sleep. Both cats are asleep on the towels I put on my bed pillows. I remove the towels when I retire. Putting your head on a pillow covered with cat hair is a poor way to start a night of sleep. The noise of the tripped toilet covers my foot noises on the carpet as I go at last to the kitchen for coffee. This is important because I am still in my walking shorts.

As I sit down in the red rocker to rest and enjoy the hot after-walk caffeine, Self compliments me. "Walking keeps you in a better condition. Today the walk seemed to be effortless for you."

"Yes, and it was painless. The over-the-counter pills are helping me replace my worn knee cartilage. I did the hill and the overpass while breathing only through my nostrils. I'm not tired, only sweaty, as I arrive home these days."

I cool down as I enjoy my coffee with the morning paper. It is a good day in spite of the early awakening. I'll probably pay for the early start by tiring in the afternoon. I wish I could develop the habit of afternoon naps. Last week I had the same early awakening scenario and I ran out of fuel in the midafternoon. I stepped on my body accelerator and walked faster while marketing in the next county. I could not find enough energy to finish. I thought my body transmission had stripped its gears. My muscles ached. I was tired. I stopped for a cup of espresso and told the server, "Put an extra shot of caffeine in it."

The smart-aleck kid asked, "Your rubber band drive ran down?"

"You bet, and I hope you have a guarantee on this stuff."

I hope my rubber band doesn't run down too quick today. I have a lot to do as I turn on the word processor.

An hour later as I take my empty cup to the kitchen I note a book I want to take Jacquie. "Self, I'm lucky."

"How so?"

"If that heart problem I had five years ago had been fatal instead of a warning, JJL would be out on a limb by herself. This way I'm around to help ease her life." I shut down the computer and notice Latte lying on her back on the sunny floor. She doesn't usually like her tummy petted, but I get in two or three strokes on this soft warm fur before she grabs my hand with her front paws, claws withdrawn. She pulls my hand so she can lick it in appreciation and love. I miss my Jacquie, but all love is not lost with these felines around to share theirs with me.

I didn't know it then but another set of cats would make life interesting as they descended upon me over the next several nights. They are beautiful but I hesitate to share their existence with my neighbors.

My neighbors will find out about them, I find.

Chapter 36

After Hours Peepshows
Early Morning Beauties

Two weeks ago I would have never known I had a backyard menagerie if my Jacquie had been home. She would nudge my ribs and say, "Wake up Don, you'll never see your TV program if you're asleep."

"I'm not asleep."

"You were snoring."

"That's to tease you. I'm listening with my eyes shut."

"Go to bed."

It's easier to take those orders than to stay awake, so I am often in bed by the middle of the evening when she is home. That is why I was missing the action in our back yard, I learn.

Before she went to the rest home she was my supervisor. Yesterday, I read of a study that found men and women switch roles at midlife. Men who are aggressive in early life moderate while docile women become assertive and assume leadership. Maybe that's what's happening to …. Self interrupts my thinking. "Don't think any further, Don. You'll get into trouble." Now living alone with the coffee cats, Latte and Mocha, I have little guidance other than Self. The cats sleep in the evening and they don't bother me. One night recently I wanted to see a British mystery at ten but I fell asleep in the recliner too soon. I awakened at one-thirty, turned off the noisy TV ads and took my bedtime medicine before going to bed.

It is then I notice Mocha, on my pillow. She is watching something on the patio. "What'cha watchin'?" I ask but she only turns her head towards me a moment before turning back to the fascination outside. I lie down beside her and I spot a dark shape. As my eyes became adjusted I too see a creature. I suffered Immaculate Conception - no, no, macular degeneration - in my right eye several years ago. Its peripheral vision supports my left eye and I have learned to adjust. What I see in the full moonlight is a very black shape with two brilliant white stripes running over its back, a skunk. It is daintily eating the cracked sunflower seed I put on the patio for ground-feeding birds. "Enjoy the sight, Mocha. You're better off viewing that cat from inside the house."

The little nocturnal fellow is busy eating with little body movement. Its erect tail is wider and longer than the animal. I am now fully awake and enjoying my backyard zoo. This is a creature of beauty in the light of the bright full moon. In a moment another skunk, equally well behaved, joins the feast. I finally go to sleep after a few more peeks out the low window at pillow level.

The next night a skunk is present again at my bedtime. Other nights I see two and three individuals feeding together. My watching continues for ten nights. One night a small opossum runs across the patio and later an immature raccoon stops to eat some peanuts.

Meanwhile, our son inspects a neighbor's house and finds a skunk in the crawl space. When the neighbor tells me about it, I ask him, "If I see skunks in my yard tonight, do you want me to call you so you can shut the opening it uses?"

"Sure!"

At one thirty-five-AM I call. "Bob, I have two skunks in my yard."

"Thanks. I'll shut the opening I found." He checks the next day and finds no skunk in his crawl space. He's happy.

Receiving a brochure on skunks I write an information sheet for my immediate neighbors, telling them Bob is taking in his birdseed at night and I will do the same. It also states, "With enough food, skunks can produce two litters a summer and opossums can produce three, so let's put away the pet food at night and not leave chattel around to provide shelter." I also report, "Arlene on the cross street set a new senior fifty-yard dash record when she came around her house and surprised a skunk." I note that several cats have been sprayed and I include several deodorizing solutions.

Since Mrs. Zur, a block east of me is upset about several evenings of odor, I take her the information sheet, but I also have an ulterior motive. "You did a good job with this, Don. Are you going to distribute it? There's a lot of concern in the neighborhood."

"No. Do you think neighbors should see it?"

"Oh, yes."

"Tell you what, Mrs. Zur, I'll print up several dozen so you can pass them out."

"Sure. I'll do it."

"Done. I'll have them at your house in an hour." I do and she is as happy as I am. She is a sociable lady and this gives her a legitimate excuse to have a quest.

I rent two traps and set them, using peanuts and sunflower seeds. I don't tell Mrs. Zur. She is a good communicator and I don't want an animal lover on her street, who sets pet food on the front porch for raccoons and other wildlife, to hear from my message carrier of my trapping at this time.

That night I go to bed shortly after midnight and am surprised to see a skunk in each trap and a third circling the traps. In a way I am happy, I guess. I had enjoyed watching those polite little fellows with great table manners, so it is no surprise that I don't sleep well during the night. I am betraying them.

Awakening at five as usual, I wait until six to call animal control. I am given the police clerk, who says the animal control lady has the day off. "Bummer, what do I do now?" I ask myself. The skunks will be sitting on bricks, in the near one-hundred-degree sun. The reflected sun can kill them. I don't want to try to pick up the traps to move them. That would be risky.

I call the Pleasanton Police. "Our two cities cooperate with a joint fire department, do you cooperate with Livermore on picking up trapped skunks?" I ask.

"No way."

"What'll I do?" I ask.

"Try calling the county department. Here's the number." Since the department isn't open this early I go to my eight o'clock meeting and call at nine upon returning.

"I have some skunks trapped and there is no animal control officer in Livermore. Will you pick them up? Please."

"No. You're in town. We just enforce the nonincorporated areas. Sorry."

"But if my neighboring animal rights activist hears the skunks died of heat and calls several TV stations, you'll get mentioned also, even if you're in the county seat twenty-five miles way."

"I'll put you through to the head of the department. Hang on." I get an answering machine that says to leave a message. I leave the same message mentioning the TV and skunks dying in the sun.

Ten minutes later I receive a call to verify my address. The man says, "I'm on my way."

"Where are you coming from?"

"The county jail." That's only five miles away. The headman called this fellow and issued the order. I am getting results.

The man from the jail arrives but his needle holder on his long stick used to inject the lethal chemical, is broken. He makes a quick round trip. He soon has the skunks under control without any odor in my yard. Before he leaves he remarks, "My boss, Tony, said to say hello to you. You were his principal in grade school."

I set the traps again and have a third skunk the next night. This time the local officer is on duty. Jacquie is spending the night, and I waken her to view the beautiful animal in the trap. As a city girl she didn't see skunks except on the highway when little beauty remained.

I comment to the officer, who is dealing with this latest animal, "My neighbor tells me there are a lot of people in the neighborhood having skunk problems."

"Yes," she replies. "A neighbor two blocks away has had me collect six or eight from his traps." She tells me that when ground was broken for a new housing/commercial area a mile away, forty skunks were found. Later, Mrs. Zur stops by to relate that another neighbor had a skunk spray in her yard last night.

The next night waking at two, I watch a skunk push into the opening of a trap beside another skunk already just inside one trap. Suddenly, the trap springs. The second trap is also successful; three skunks in two traps. In six nights I trap eight skunks. The last one is a big male, the largest the control officer has seen. By the end of two weeks eleven skunks have been trapped. The next morning I see another of these black and whites three blocks away as I start my before-dawn walk, and find that another has eaten some peanuts in the shell leaving the hull ends.

I receive a call from a neighbor who has had odors for four nights in a row. She too will trap. It seems with birdseed, cat and dog food and ponds in urban backyards, the wildlife is doing better than if it had to depend on bugs and beetles in the dry rural areas.

I've become known as the skunk man of the area, and word of my results spreads in the neighborhood. At a city meeting about developing the field to the north, a neighbor said, "Development will move wildlife into town. Larsen on Lincoln has already caught a number of skunks." The neighbors who are present set up a cheer.

I also hear some interesting stories of skunk adaptation to our human scene. "Don, I heard a noise in my kitchen and went to check on it. Our cats were on the counter with backs hunched, tails splayed and looking down. On the floor was a skunk eating from their cat dish." It had entered through the pet door in the kitchen door. Another said, "While duck hunting I stepped on a dead skunk in a harvested field. In town I put my foot in a cafe toilet and flushed repeatedly, but could not remove the odor. Then someone told me to go to the store and get a gallon of catsup. After putting my foot in the catsup there was no longer any smell."

I decide to continue to trap. I see footprints on the south side of the house and catch a skunk there. The next night I look out the window to see if there is any action. A skunk is just leaving the side of the trap to go out under the gate. It had dug under the trap, allowing the peanuts and sunflower seeds to fall through the trap where they could be reached. The animal had no need to enter the trap.

"You had better continue trapping another week," Self suggests, "Your neighbors have given you enough money to cover the trap rental costs."

I return to the rental store, "Gary," I say to the owner, who attended the middle school when I was the vice-principal, "I'm considering renting one of the traps a third week. Would you treat me like Safeway sometimes does, rent one and get one free? I already owe you fifty-eight dollars."

He thought a moment and surprised me. "No. Take 'em both and I'll charge you fifty-eight dollars and tax. No rent this week."

"Thanks." The rate of catch is slowing as the population declines.

However, the following week my total take rises to thirteen in almost three weeks. I hear a neighbor three blocks east has trapped one also. That brings the total to twenty-three in our small neighborhood, one block times four.

This morning's catch is a very lively smaller animal. The control officer does receive a spray, the second time that's happened with my thirteen skunks. It is only a matter of minutes until my phone begins to ring. "Don, did you get another skunk? I smelled one a few minutes ago," a talkative neighbor asks. She becomes very upset about the odor. I find the odor not unpleasant if it is not too strong.

My rental time is up tomorrow. The animal control officer offers me a city trap if I want to continue. I enjoyed watching these beautiful and well-mannered animals in the moonlight for the ten nights before I began trapping. If humans had not coaxed them into the neighborhood with pet food and water, they would still be alive. The extra food may have been enough to create several extra litters. Apparently the only enemies the skunk has are the auto and the great horned owl. We seldom see one of these delightful, nocturnal birds. There is only one local pair and it lives three miles to the east. They probably find enough skunks without coming to our corner of town.

In another day or two I make an important catch, but it is not a skunk.

Chapter 37

Oh No! Not Again!
Will We Learn To Avoid Calling 911?

It is not what I had planned. Far from it! I am visiting JJL this evening and everything is going well. The San Francisco Giants are ahead and she is feeling good. It is time for me to tell her goodbye as the closing hour is upon us.

"Don, help me to the bathroom before you go."

"No problem." The problem is not going to the bathroom; it's coming from it. To be explicit, the problem occurs as she is rising from the stool.

"Don," she announces, "I'm getting lightheaded. Hold me!" Then she faints, half-standing and half-bent over. I'm prepared to assist at all times but when the moment arrives, it's a problem.

Self asks, rather surprised, "How are you going to revive her if it takes both hands to hold her from falling?" There is little room and my initial hold is not very secure.

"Today has been tiring. I'm not feeling very strong myself," I reply.

"Jam her against the wall with your hip. You can hold her up a moment that way until we think of something," Self says in an almost reactionary and supervisory manner. "Then maybe we can ease her to the floor."

I reply, "I don't have enough strength for that, I might drop her. How can I revive her if I have my hands full and I'm weakening?" Complications. I wish there were a call button in this bathroom.

"Don, you're asking more questions than you're answering. Think."

Then I have an inspiration. Instead of yelling at the top of my lungs for help and frightening all the elderly residents in the home, I will use my cell phone to call Sergeant Sue. She's in the kitchen.

"There might be a problem," Self moans. "She's on her cellular most of the day. You'll get a busy signal. Good luck, Don." I am already calling her number.

"HelloChateauLivermore.ThisisSuespeaking.HowmayIhelpyou?" Oh, that lady can talk faster than I can listen. I can't understand her; at least I know I have the right number.

"Sue, this is Don. Jacquie is down in the bathroom. I need help, now!'

"What? Whatdidyousay? IsthisDon? I'll be right there."

She runs down the hall with a wheelchair and comes into the bathroom. Will we have a big problem when we're able to revive JJL? Sue calls her manager, who is a nurse, and I call the advice nurse of our HMO. I then call 911.

The firehouse is two blocks away. I hope the crew with paramedics is there rather than exercising the engine or taking a break at the ice cream store two miles away. We get JJL into her wheelchair and take blood pressure and blood sugar levels. "What's next?" Self asks.

"We'll soon find out what to do." Forgetting I'm talking to Self, I answer aloud. "Won't we?"

"I hope so," Sergeant Sue answers as she starts down the hall. "I'd better get the front door unlocked and open for the firemen." She keeps the door locked for security reasons and asks, "Who's there?" whenever the doorbell sounds. She is good at looking out windows to see if she recognizes cars parked out front.

"Who's coming?" my wife asks, more alert now.

"The 911 folks," I answer. I check the blood pressure reading I've taken, which is acceptable.

"They weren't at the ice cream parlor," Self says. "I hear them coming around the corner."

Moments later Sue is leading them into the bedroom.

One look at Jacquie and the lead fireman says, "Let's get her out of the wheelchair and lay her on the carpet. We need to take her vitals." In a moment he is listening with his stethoscope as another of the crew is wrapping a blood pressure cuff on Jacquie's arm.

As she begins responding to the questions a crewman is reading from his clipboard, the fellows from an ambulance arrive and take over the questioning and the checking of the vital signs. They snap the gurney into position and load her on, preparing to leave for the emergency room.

As the firemen are gathering their gear, one asks me if I remember him. "My dad was Danny, a barber, and you had me when you were vice-principal at Junction Avenue School. We used to live near you on South M Street."

"A long time ago. Yeah, I remember but wouldn't have recognized you. Maybe you didn't come into my office enough for us to become very well acquainted."

"I just managed to avoid trips to the office. I'm retiring in several months."

"Well, thanks for getting here so promptly, and for your help. I'd better head for Walnut Creek and the hospital. I'd like to be there to explain things to the admitting nurse. My wife doesn't remember too much about her problem. Bye, and thanks again."

It's about seven-thirty. I tell Sue I will call her when I find out anything. "If they don't keep her overnight, I'll take her home and bring her out here in the morning."

"Please call, Mr. Larsen, and let me know how she is." This little guardian is very protective of her charges. Since I have my cell phone it will be easy to report to her. As I go out the door, she reminds me, "Drive carefully, Mr. Larsen. Be safe!"

It's a good thing I'm there to help admit Jacquie. I'm learning more about her dementia as we live these months. "Tell me what happened," the emergency room doctor asks us and I repeat what I told the admitting nurse. "We'll read her vitals and watch her," this man says with what appears to be a genuine interest. In a quarter of an hour he is back from checking other emergency room patients, and asks, "Why are you taking neurotin?"

"To prevent my migraines from coming back."

"It helps?"

'You'd better believe it," she replies with her strongest voice so far.

On a later visit he asks, "How soon did you get results after starting to take it?"

"The headaches stopped after the first pill and I haven't had but one migraine in the six months since. It's a miracle drug, Doctor."

"I have some patients with migraines. I think I'd better investigate this and consider using it," he says. Again, he returns to the ER nerve center and the concerns of another patient.

Jacquie is resting and we guess we will be going home soon. I called the sergeant not long ago. In time the doctor returns to say he doesn't think she had a stroke or a heart attack and he is dismissing her. "Set up an ER follow-up appointment with your doctor as soon as possible. Good night." We like him as a person and also as a doctor.

"It's always good to be dismissed home rather than assigned to a ward room when in the ER," Self whispers as I wheel her to the car in the HMO's wheelchair. I repeat that thought to her as I help her into the car after steadying her long enough for an embrace and a kiss.

"I love you, Don. I'm so sorry I ruined your evening. You haven't had anything to eat either."

"There's food at home." The commute traffic has long since passed and it is a clear full-moon night. We enjoy the ride. She has a hand on my knee and I have my right arm around her shoulders. "I'm glad I was there to catch you," I tell her and she squeezes my knee one more time.

She did not get any medicine in the ER, but she gets some when we go into our house. The cats are waiting. Latte licks JJL's extended hand while Mocha squeaked several soft Mewws to her. My Jacquie forgets what has happened and welcomes them to bed with her before I get my late dinner. Before I come to bed I call the HMO's twenty-four-hour number and set up an appointment with Dr. Banda. She has an opening near noon tomorrow and it's assigned to JJL. Things are falling into place for Jacquie, it seems.

Jacquie gets to sleep in and we have a leisurely breakfast before I dress her for the appointment. "She's feeling fine, it appears," Self says. I concur.

"What's happening?" Doctor Banda asks. A quick review of yesterday's events and the results on the main computer don't seem to worry our doctor. "She raised her hands quickly to shampoo recently. Jacquie, you quickly exerted yourself to stand yesterday and that is straining your system. Remember, it was a quick exertion several other times that has caused her trouble. I have said the word quickly several times. You must take time to stand up or change body positions. Remember that, Jacquie. I like you, but I don't want to see you under these conditions. Telling you and warning you is all I can do. You have to change your habits, Jacquie!"

Hearing her name several times in a row makes a point with her, but will she remember what she has learned?

It is hard to change decades of habit and practice. She falls again in the near future. I came home one day to hear a message on the answering machine, "Mr.Larsenyour Jacquieshefall againatthree this afternoon. Canyoucome?" The message is only thirty minutes old and Sue is excited. I leave immediately.

"What happened?" I ask as she lies in bed. "Are you hurt?"

"I got up to use the commode, I guess. I wakened on the floor between it and the bed. I don't remember falling. Then I guess I walked into the bathroom without my walker. No, I'm not hurt."

"Lucky you!"

"Sylvia heard what was happening and used her call button for Sue."

"That's why I chose a double room for you, so you can have some help if you need it." Sue has five other ladies to care for, and I figure I can care for JJL on weekends by myself: a one-to-one ratio. How wrong I am. Last Sunday I awakened before dawn and was enjoying coffee in the red rocker when I heard a thump, thump. I figured it was the cats starting the day with a chase game over the bed. I was wrong.

"Don. Don," JJL cried. "Help me up. I've fallen." It never takes me long to enter a room following that message. I found her sitting on the floor with her back against the lavatory cabinet. "I had to go to the bathroom I guess." I lifted her with little help from her. She had a pain below the right breast but spent the day watching a ballgame on TV. As I dress her for bed at the Chateau that evening, we noticed a silver-dollar-sized purple spot where the soreness was.

The following evening when I arrive at the Chateau, she tells me she couldn't get comfortable for sleep and has a bruise on her little toe. "Will I have to have bars on the side of my bed to keep me in it so I don't fall?" The falls are occurring almost at regular intervals. When she is asked, "Do you remember falling?" she always answers, no.

"Don, I notice you're becoming a podiatrist. Do you have a license?" Self chides me on the way home from my evening visit with Jacquie.

"Seems that way. I knew it was necessary to cut the children's nails when they were little, but having to care for four sets to care for in my septuagenarian years surprises me." It's JJL's set last night and I'm overdue on the two cats' forty nails. Mocha was kneading my back in bed this morning and her claws are too sharp.

"You'll have to put on your heavy overalls or put a heavy towel on your lap to do the felines' paws," Self reminds me. "Latte's more accepting of the clipping but Mocha engages her four paws instant reverse."

"They're getting better, Self; JJL said a podiatrist charges fifty dollars to come to the home to cut a lady's ten nails. At that rate I'm responsible for three hundred dollars' worth of clipping when you include mine. That would buy me a lot of hamburgers. I guess I'm worth something after all."

With JJL at the Chateau, I'm relieved of the constant strain of caring for her, and I should be in excellent health, I think. That is not the case. One day I am delivering reports also dropping off newsletters in one of the far corners of our area when I notice I am faint and beginning to sweat. Coming out of one real estate office, I wonder if I can reach the car before I collapse. I look around to see if there is anyone to steady me but no one is near. I manage to drive several blocks and ask myself if I should stop at the emergency room, which is just a short distance away. A wave of lightheadedness sweeps over me, but I remain alert enough to park in the emergency lot and check myself into the unit.

A CAT scan, an EKG and a blood draw don't turn up a problem. My blood sugar is low and the blood pressure a little high. "See your doctor next week," is the advice I receive. The next day Dr. Banda obtains the same readings and changes my blood pressure prescription.

A day or two later and I can begin to tell the difference. This morning I do my walk after a slow start, but I have an extra shot of caffeine in my coffee to hit my stride. This artificial burst of energy wears off and I awaken after the ball game is over wondering which team won. I have a number of irons in my fires, and I believe part of my problem is stress. I must learn to recognize it quicker.

Another factor may be this business of aging. I may not have the horsepower I once had under my hood. Lately I have been sleeping only five or six hours a night and that bothers me enough to check it. A little research tells me that older folks don't need as much sleep and Dr. Banda concurs. I fall asleep early and waken in the middle of the night. Is there a way to set my body clock back several hours? I'm adjusting to the fact that my mind refreshes before my body by doing a lot of thinking and planning before arising.

I am about ready to apologize to myself about a habit I'm developing. I find it refreshing to take my cup of coffee to the red rocker before dressing and sit in the dark just doing nothing. This is becoming one of my favorite times of the day. The cats often join me to get some petting and purr their love to me. Yesterday I made the mistake of sitting in the recliner rather than the rocker. I had my feet raised and Latte let me know I should put the lap robe in place. When she didn't jump onto my lap I remembered she wants to nap on the green side. She's leapt immediately onto the robe once I turned the green side up.

After coffee I go to the computer and am joined by Mocha, who competes with the monitor for my attention. Then it's time to dress and start my walk. I hear a sound and find Latte has jumped onto the seat of the porch swing in the office and the swinging seat is the source of the noise. This tidy cat is busily grooming her rear right foot while swinging.

This week shifted into overdrive, it seems. I am skipping a marketing meeting to go to an Eldercare meeting about dementia. The admission price is right, and it's time I know more about this condition that is to stay with Jacquie and me from now on. The group is small and we don't talk much about dementia in general. Two of the group have mothers with severe cases of Alzheimer's Disease, and the discussion centers on this form of dementia. I come away feeling grateful that this isn't Jacquie's problem. I will give to the next Alzheimer's fund drive. That's bad stuff. Unfortunately, it attacks older people generally and our population is becoming older.

It is midmorning on Saturday when I collect JJL and her gear for our weekend date. Sergeant Sue has more clothes than Jacquie'll need packed with her insulin gear and medicines. I take the walker and leave the wheelchair as she gets so little exercise at the home. I'll hold her arm at all times as we walk. I forgot to go to the Farmer's Market in Livermore Thursday so I wonder if the kettle corn man will be in Pleasanton today. JJL appears to be up to going to several stalls with me. It will be exercise for her and an interesting change of pace from the weeklong diet of TV and the routine of the rest home.

I don't have to coax her out of the car. She unbuckles the seat belt and we start investigating the stalls. "I am amazed at the varieties of breads," she says as she chooses a French cheese bread. Then she finds a Cornish pasty, the kind that is mentioned in several of the British mysteries we are reading. She asks the vendor, "Please give me one without onions." Next she buys individual rhubarb pies and jam. The vegetables are not only beautiful, many are unusual. She talks a lot to stall owners, a most unusual activity for her. I'm surprised she wants to keep walking and looking. We overdo it and she becomes weak. A chair is found, and after resting we buy our giant bag of kettle corn.

The animal adoption agency finds it wise to bring their dogs and cats to an adjoining park to take advantage of the crowds at the market. I am surprised when my wife says, "Don, lets go see the cats." What a variety of cats and kittens they have for adoption. A rather large Manx Siamese catches our eye. "Look at her beautiful light throat coloring and her large expressive eyes." After I place Jacquie in the car I decide to adopt this cat, who is called Mickey. I'm not sure why we need three cats; however, the two we have are certainly great for JJL's well being. Perhaps a third one, if as loving as I think Mickey is, will be that much better for Jacquie's wellbeing.

"You're thinking about your own wishes, Don," Self insists.

I don't have enough cash and the agency is not prepared to take a credit card, so I start walking the block or two to the bank. The trip is a ten-block journey, I find, in spite on being told it's just around the corner. Returning with the cash, I'm amazed at all the paperwork and all the promises I must agree to before becoming Mickey's guardian.

But she isn't ours yet. There's another act to follow. A volunteer takes her from her pen to put her into a cardboard carrying case, and she objects with all four paws. She runs up his arm, across his shoulders and down his side to land in rapid four-paw drive. She runs down the fence line with several volunteers in pursuit until she comes to the corner of the dog adoption area and stops. The lady who has been her foster mother is present and soon retrieves the frightened fleeing feline. With the aid of many hands the cat is boxed, at least for a few minutes.

I place the carrier on JJL's lap and start to drive home. "I want to see our kitty," JJL says, as she opens one of the holding tabs on the cardboard carrier to peek inside. Mickey is an opportunist. Seeing a crack develop, she pushes her head against the slightly parted lids and then, with her tremendous power dialed to max, she floorboards her exit. She is over the seats before Jacquie can admire her. Fortunately, all the windows are closed. Mickey finds the deck by the rear windshield to give both a good view and an area of comfort. She rides the ten miles home there.

Having witnessed two escapes, I use the remote control to shut the garage door before considering opening a car door.

Turning to Jacquie, I voice a new set of concerns. "Why don't we give her a coffee name like the other two?"

"Like what?"

"I don't know. Cappuccino?"

"No. That's too hard to say. You'll have to do better'n that."

"Cuppa' Joe's not any better. I'll keep thinkin'. Right now we've got the problem of introducing her to the other cats. They'll not be happy, I'll bet. I had to explain to the adoption agency how I'll do this. Oh, I'll need to take her to Dr. Bird next week to have an identity chip placed under the skin between her shoulders, like Latte and Mocha."

I am able to carry Mickey as far as the dining room. Then she digs several claws into me for leverage; she bolts to the floor and dashes into the bedroom towards the covers hanging off the bed. It is an adjustable bed and soon she is in the box under the folding platform. The two resident cats see her and go into a quiet 911 alert. Tails, ears and noses are trying to gather details about the interloper.

"Now what are you going to do?" Jacquie asks.

"I'll not interfere. They need time to adjust themselves. It may take several days to get acquainted." I bring Mickey out, but she quickly runs under my desk in the studio, out of reach. "I'll put some water and food near her and a box of litter. She lets me pet her and she licks my hand," I report to Jacquie.

Latte and Mocha avoid the new cat. They look at her from a distance now and then, and a few growls are exchanged, but they ignore Mickey for the most part. We go to bed but leave a light on.

In the morning, I arise and go searching for Mickey. She's nowhere – I've lost her again.

"How's our new kitty?" JJL asks when she wakens.

"I don't know. I can't find her. Dawn will be lighting the house better soon and I'll look again."

That is enough to bring my wife from bed. She starts to hunt also. Now I have two females to focus on. I need to find Mickey and watch that my Jacquie doesn't fall as she tries to bend over to peek under furniture. She has enough trouble keeping her balance just walking.

Before long I find Mickey on the towels in the lower part of the linen closet. The doors were slightly ajar last night. That is the first hint her specialty is opening cabinet doors.

She doesn't want to come out, so I talk to her and let her lick my hand. She is amenable to petting and scratching below her ears. I talk to her and introduce myself. The negotiations suddenly deteriorate and she hisses. "Why are you hissing?" I ask. I then see that Latte has heard me talking and has arrived to check the proceedings. She's invaded Mickey's defensive territory.

For several hours, with food and water and a litter pan near, we visit our newest, petting her and talking, giving calm reassurances. JJL is worried she'll not have a chance to become acquainted with Mickey before she goes back to the Chateau.

During halftime of the Sunday afternoon football game we look up and see that Mickey is now venturing into the main part of the house. She is very careful. We sit still and talk to her. Gradually, with a lot of false starts and rapid tail motion, she approaches JJL and rubs against my wife's hand. She's purring. She spends the next several hours exploring and I do a lot of brushing of Latte's coat as I assure her that Mickey's going to be a friend. "Just take your time getting acquainted," I advise. Mocha is across the room with attention on the drama.

After taking my wife to the home and putting her to bed, I arrive back at the house to see that each of the cats has found a different place to begin their early evening naps.

I sleep well and longer than usual. Now where are the cats? I wonder. "The original ones are in their usual places, but where is Mickey?" Self asks. This business of cat hunting several times a day is making life interesting. And then I spot her. She has found a medium-sized basket on the counter above where she was sleeping on towels and she is curled inside. Her eyes open and she recognizes me. She is ready to lick my proffered hand and accept some petting and conversation. All is well. I can start on my walk.

Quick Order Form

Fax order: 1 800 481-7638

Telephone Orders: Toll free 1 800 481-7638
   Have your credit card ready.

Email orders: donlarsen@activebooks.com

Postal Orders: Active Books, 358 Lincoln Ave., Livermore, CA, 94550

On-line Orders: www.active-books.com

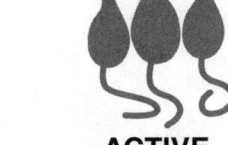
ACTIVE BOOKS

❏ **Please send the following books:**

_____ $_____.____

I may return any books for full refund, no questions

Sales tax: Please add 08.25% for books shipped to CA   ($_____.____)

Shipping: Flat $2.00 Active Books will cover the balance $2.00

                                                              Total $_____.____

❏ **Please send other FREE information.**

Send to:

Name _____

Address _____

City_____ State_____ Zip _____

Telephone _____

Email _____

Payment:

❏ Check; ❏ Credit card; ❏ Visa; ❏ MasterCard; ❏ Discovery

Card number: _____ Expires: ___/___/___

Name on card: _____

Quick Order Form

Fax order: 1 800 481-7638
Telephone Orders: Toll free 1 800 481-7638
  Have your credit card ready.
Email orders: donlarsen@activebooks.com
Postal Orders: Active Books, 358 Lincoln Ave., Livermore, CA, 94550
On-line Orders: www.active-books.com

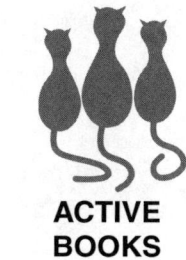
ACTIVE BOOKS

❏ **Please send the following books:**

_____ $_____.____

I may return any books for full refund, no questions
Sales tax: Please add 08.25% for books shipped to CA   ($_____.____)
Shipping: Flat $2.00 Active Books will cover the balance $2.00
                                                      Total $_____.____

❏ **Please send other FREE information.**

Send to:

Name _____

Address _____

City_____ State_____ Zip _____

Telephone _____

Email _____

Payment:

❏ Check; ❏ Credit card; ❏ Visa; ❏ MasterCard; ❏ Discovery

Card number: _____ Expires: ___/___/___

Name on card: _____